Understanding Breast Cancer

With Orthodox and Alternative Treatments

Preface

I have written this book so that the patients suffering from Breast cancer can understand the disease in detail and choose a suitable treatment for them. This book provides detailed information about the clinical symptoms, complications, diagnosis, staging and treatments. In the last 15 years there has been considerable research and progress in the field of clinical studies, etiology, pathology, diagnosis and treatment of Breast cancer. Today we have new medicines, which work in a better way.

In this book, I have written in detail about Orthodox and Alternative Treatment (Budwig Protocol, which is the best alternative treatment and gives authentic success). Patient can carefully select the right treatment for him. This book has up to date information.

Dr. O.P.Verma

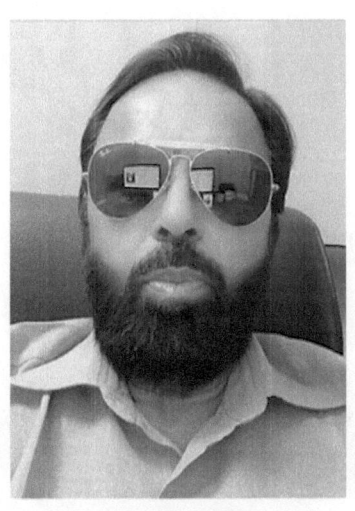

Written by
Dr. O.P.Verma
M.B.B.S., M.R.S.H. (London)
Budwig Wellness
7-B-43, Mahaveer Nagar III, Kota (Raj.)
+919460816360

Table of Content

Understanding Breast Cancer..1

Anatomy & Physiology of the Breast.....................................3

U.S. Breast Cancer Statistics...7

Risk factors for Developing Breast Cancer..........................10

Breast Cancer Types and Subtypes..11

Breast Cancer Clinical Presentation...16

Workup 19

Breast Cancer Screening...20

Mammogram 21

Ultrasound...22

MRI..23

Positron Emission Tomography...23

Scintimammography..24

Breast Biopsy..24

Lab tests for hormone receptors 28

HER2/neu Test..30

Stages of breast cancer 33

Treatment..37

Surgery 42

Chemotherapy..48

Radiation Therapy...55

Hormone Therapy..62

Targeted Therapy..68

Breast cancer prevention 75

Guide to Breast Self-Examination..*78*

Managing Finances When You Have Breast Cancer **81**

Breast Cancer in Young Women **86**

Can I Refuse Breast Cancer Treatment?...**96**

Alternative cancer treatments **102**

Chemotherapy Doesn't Cure Cancer – It Causes It!........................*102*

Laetrile (Vitamin B-17) Therapy..**104**

The Gerson Therapy **109**

Simoncini's Baking Soda Cancer Treatment.................................**112**

Best Alternative Treatment - Budwig Protocol **113**

Prime Cause of Cancer **116**

Otto Warburg   Biography...*116*

Prime cause of Cancer...*118*

Dr. Johanna Budwig - Biography & Science.................................**120**

Budwig Protocol..**127**

Budwig Diet...*128*

Precautions..*135*

Prohibitions of Budwig Protocol...*137*

Few Desserts recipes by Dr. Budwig...*139*

ELDI oils *141*

Coffee Enema *145*

Epsom bath *148*

Soda bicarb bath *149*

Sun Therapy..*149*

Oil-Protein Diet while travelling *150*

Making Quark *152*

Making Cottage Cheese *152*

Buckwheat..*153*

Energy Healing *155*

How long should you take this protocol? *156*

How do I recognize a good Flax seed oil?.....................................*157*

Questions and Answers...**159**

Budwig Diet & Protocol - In Brief..**161**

Lothar Hirneise **164**

Interview of Dr. Johanna Budwig **169**

Sun, Photons and Electrons..**177**

Electrons...*177*

The sun's energy and man as an antenna.....................................*178*

Fats Syndrome..*180*

The electrons as resonance system *182*

Visualization - Path to wellness...**186**

Unresolved trauma or shock **191**

Breast Cancer always follows Psychological Trauma *192*

Testimonials of Budwig Protocol **196**

The Budwig Diet quotes **204**

My Books...**213**

Understanding Breast Cancer

Worldwide, breast cancer is the most frequently diagnosed life-threatening cancer in women. In many less-developed countries, it is the leading cause of cancer death in women; in developed countries, however, it has been surpassed by lung cancer as a cause of cancer death in women. In the United States, breast cancer accounts for 30% of all cancers in women and is second only to lung cancer as a cause of cancer deaths.

Many early breast cancers are asymptomatic; pain or discomfort is not usually a symptom of breast cancer. Breast cancer is sometimes first detected as an abnormality on a mammogram before it is felt by the patient or healthcare provider.

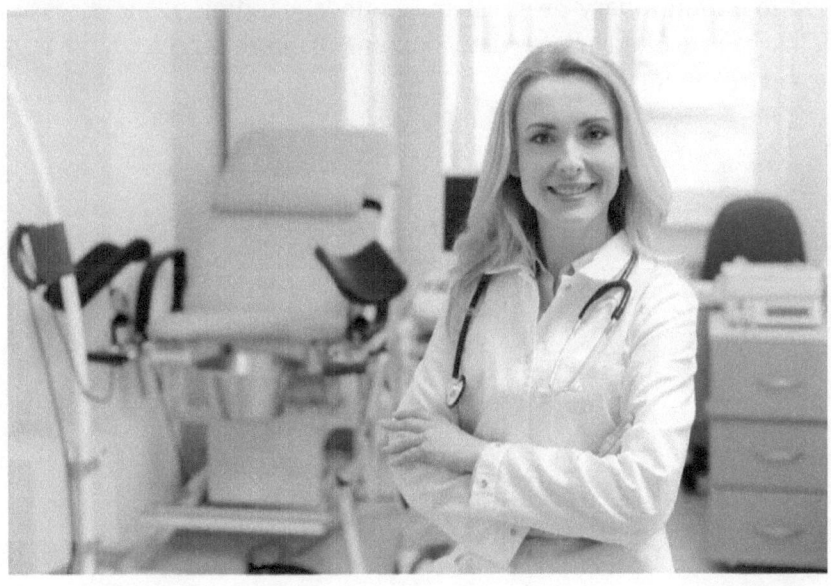

The general approach to evaluation of breast cancer has become formalized as triple assessment: clinical examination, imaging (usually mammography, ultrasonography, or both), and needle biopsy. Increased public awareness and improved screening have led to earlier diagnosis, at stages amenable to complete surgical resection and curative therapies. Improvements in therapy and screening have led to improved prognosis for women diagnosed with breast cancer.

Surgery and radiation therapy, along with adjuvant hormone or chemotherapy when indicated, are now considered primary treatment for breast cancer. For many patients with low-risk early-stage breast cancer, surgery with local radiation is curative.

Adjuvant breast cancer therapies are designed to treat micrometastatic disease or breast cancer cells that have escaped the breast and regional lymph nodes but do not yet have an established identifiable metastasis. Depending on the model of risk reduction, adjuvant therapy has been estimated to be responsible for 35-72% of the decrease in mortality.

Over the past 3 decades, extensive breast cancer research has led to extraordinary progress in the understanding of the disease. This has resulted in the development of more targeted and less toxic treatments.

Anatomy & Physiology of the Breast

The breast is an organ whose special function is the production of milk for lactation (breast feeding). The female adult breast contains 14–18 irregular lactiferous lobules, where milk is produced, which connect to ducts that lead out to the nipple. Most cancers of the breast arise from the cells which form the lobules and terminal ducts. These lobules and ducts are spread throughout the background fibrous tissue and adipose tissue (fat) that make up the majority of the breast. The male breast structure is nearly identical to the female breast, except that the male breast tissue lacks the specialized lobules, since there is no physiologic need for milk production by males.

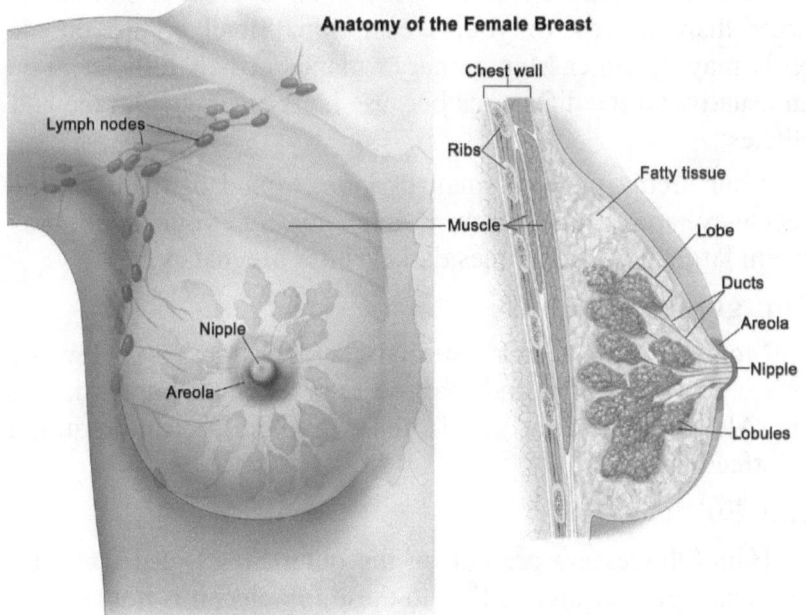

Anatomy of the Female Breast

Anatomically, the adult breast sits atop the pectoralis major muscle ("pec" = the chest muscle), which is atop the ribcage. The breast tissue extends horizontally (side-to-side) from the edge of the sternum (the firm flat bone in the middle of the chest) out to the midaxillary line (the center of the axilla, or underarm). A tail of breast tissue called the "axillary tail of Spence" extend into the underarm area. This is important because a breast cancer can develop in this axillary tail, even though it might not seem to be located within the actual breast.

The breast tissue is encircled by a thin layer of connective tissue called fascia. The deep layer of this fascia sits immediately atop the pectoralis muscle, and the superficial layer sits just under the skin. The skin covering the breast is similar to skin elsewhere on the body and has similar sweat glands, hair follicles, and other features. A clinician will examine the skin in addition to the breast tissue itself when performing a breast exam.

Areola

Surrounding the nipple is your areola, an area of skin that is darker than the rest of your breast skin. Small bumps on the areola may be either Montgomery's glands or hair follicles. You can usually tell the difference because hairs emerge from the hair follicles.

Your areola may be small or large, round or oval. During pregnancy, areolas may grow in diameter, and your areola may remain larger (and sometimes darker) after pregnancy.

Montgomery Glands

Montgomery glands are special glands that lie just below the surface of your areola and may be seen as small bumps in the skin. Also called areolar glands, these provide lubrication during breastfeeding.

Hair Follicles

Hair follicles are present on the outer breast, especially on the surface of your areola. Due to these follicles, it is not unusual to have a few hairs growing on the surface of your areola or breast skin. If these are bothersome, carefully trim them. Pulling them out with tweezers can be painful and may open the way to infections.

4

Sulcus (of the Breast)

At the intersection of the areola and the rising edge of the nipple is a fold called the sulcus. It may be a smooth curve of skin, or it may look like a wrinkle. Inverted nipples may hide within the sulcus while retracted nipples may pull in at the sulcus line.

Muscles and Ligaments of the Breast

Nipples are held erect by small, smooth muscles that respond to signals from your autonomic nervous system (the "unconscious" nervous system over which you do not have voluntary control). Nipple erection can be caused by cold temperature or stimulation. Even though nipples can respond to sensual caresses, they are not considered sex organs.

Cooper's Ligaments

Cooper's Ligaments form a hammock for your breast tissue to keep its shape. These ligaments run from tissue in your collarbone and chest wall throughout the breast and up to the areola skin. With age, these ligaments often stretch, leading to the popular slang term "Coops droop."

Blood Supply & Lymph Nodes

The blood supply from the breast comes primarily from the internal mammary artery, which runs underneath the main breast tissue. The blood supply provides nutrients, such as oxygen, to the breast tissue. The lymphatic vessels of the breast flow in the opposite direction of the blood supply and drain into lymph nodes. It is through these lymphatic vessels that breast cancers metastasize or spread to lymph nodes. Most lymphatic vessels flow to the axillary (underarm) lymph nodes, while a smaller number of lymphatic vessels flow to internal mammary lymph nodes located deep to the breast. Knowledge of this lymphatic drainage is important, because when a breast cancer metastasizes, it usually involves the first lymph node in the chain of lymph nodes. This is called the "sentinel lymph node," and a surgeon

5

may remove this lymph node to check for metastases in a patient with breast cancer.

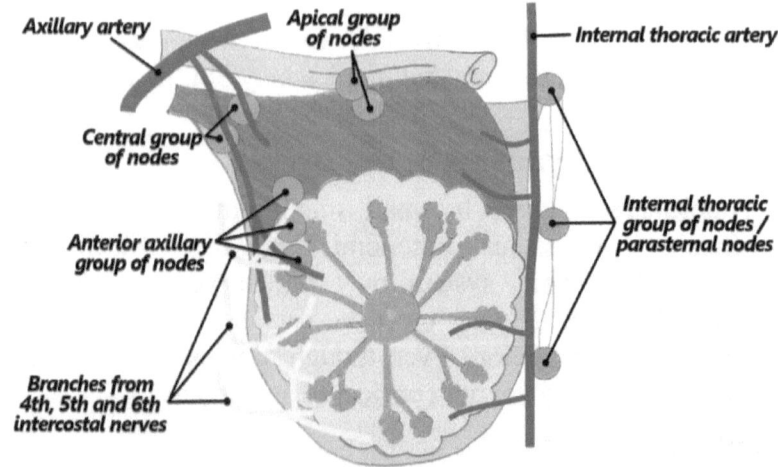

Axillary artery

Apical group of nodes

Internal thoracic artery

Central group of nodes

Internal thoracic group of nodes / parasternal nodes

Anterior axillary group of nodes

Branches from 4th, 5th and 6th intercostal nerves

Many additional changes are seen in the breast tissue during pregnancy and lactation due to the changes in hormones during those times.

U.S. Breast Cancer Statistics

- About 1 in 8 U.S. women (about 12%) will develop invasive breast cancer over the course of her lifetime. One in every 14 women in India has this cancer.

- In 2019, an estimated 268,600 new cases of invasive breast cancer are expected to be diagnosed in women in the U.S., along with 62,930 new cases of non-invasive (in situ) breast cancer.

- About 2,670 new cases of invasive breast cancer are expected to be diagnosed in men in 2019. A man's lifetime risk of breast cancer is about 1 in 883.

- Breast cancer incidence rates in the U.S. began decreasing in the year 2000, after increasing for the previous two decades. They dropped by 7% from 2002 to 2003 alone. **One theory is that this decrease was partially due to the reduced use of hormone replacement therapy (HRT) by women after the results of a large study called the Women's Health Initiative were published in 2002. These results suggested a connection between HRT and increased breast cancer risk.**

- About 41,760 women in the U.S. are expected to die in 2019 from breast cancer, though death rates have been decreasing since 1989. Women under 50 have experienced larger decreases. These decreases are thought to be the result of treatment advances, earlier detection through screening, and increased awareness.

- For women in the U.S., breast cancer death rates are higher than those for any other cancer, besides lung cancer.

- Besides skin cancer, breast cancer is the most commonly diagnosed cancer among American women. In 2019, it's estimated that about 30% of newly diagnosed cancers in women will be breast cancers.

- In women under 45, breast cancer is more common in African-American women than white women. Overall, African-American women are more likely to die of breast cancer. For Asian, Hispanic, and Native-American women, the risk of developing and dying from breast cancer is lower.

- As of January 2019, there are more than 3.1 million women with a history of breast cancer in the U.S. This includes women currently being treated and women who have finished treatment.

- A woman's risk of breast cancer nearly doubles if she has a first-degree relative (mother, sister or daughter) who has been diagnosed with breast cancer. Less than 15% of women who get breast cancer have a family member diagnosed with it.

- About 5-10% of breast cancers can be linked to gene mutations inherited from one's mother or father. Mutations in the BRCA1 and BRCA2 genes are the most common. On average, women with a BRCA1 mutation have up to a 72% lifetime risk of developing breast cancer. For women with a BRCA2 mutation, the risk is 69%. Breast cancer that is positive for the BRCA1 or BRCA2 mutations tends to develop more often in younger women. An increased ovarian cancer risk is also associated with these genetic mutations. In men, BRCA2 mutations are associated with a lifetime breast cancer risk of about 6.8%; BRCA1 mutations are a less frequent cause of breast cancer in men.

- About 85% of breast cancers occur in women who have no family history of breast cancer. These occur due to genetic mutations that happen as a result of the aging process and life in general, rather than inherited mutations.

- The most significant risk factors for breast cancer are gender (being a woman) and age (growing older).
- The American Cancer Society estimates that 1.4 million women have this cancer every year in the world.

Incidence

Over the last 25 years, the incidence of breast cancer has increased, mainly due to changes in dietary habits, better diagnostic modalities, changes in age of reproduction and lack of exercise. In the world, the prevalence of cancer has increased, but after this, there has been a decrease in mortality in developed countries. This disease can occur to men too.

The incidence of different types of breast cancer is as follows.

- Infiltrating ductal carcinoma is the most common and has a 75% rate.
- The rate of lobular carcinoma in situ is 2.8%.
- Infiltrating Lobular Carcinoma rate is equivalent to 15% of Infiltrating ductal carcinoma.
- The rate of tubular carcinoma is 1-2%.
- Papillary carcinoma occurs in older women and its rate is 1-2%.
- Paget's disease rate is 1-4% and it is higher in the sixth decade of age.

Risk factors for Developing Breast Cancer

Weight: Studies have found that the chance of getting breast cancer is higher in post-menopausal women who have not used menopausal hormone therapy and who are significantly overweight compared to peers who are of a healthy weight.

Smoking: Researchers at the American Cancer Society found an increased risk for breast cancer among women who smoke, especially those who started to smoke before having their first child.

Alcohol: The National Cancer Institute reports that over 100 studies document an increased risk of breast cancer associated with alcohol consumption.

Inactive Lifestyle: Women who are physically inactive throughout life may have an increased risk of breast cancer.

Breast Cancer Types and Subtypes

Most of us tend to think of breast cancer as a single disease, but research continues to prove otherwise. In addition to the different types of breast cancer, there are a number of subtypes of the disease. The type and subtype of a breast cancer, identified in a pathology report following surgery, gives a cancer care team the information they need to develop a plan that is most appropriate for successfully treating a specific type and subtype of a breast cancer.

Breast Cancer Types

If your doctor suspects breast cancer, it's worth getting to know the different types now, so you have a basis of understanding should a diagnosis prove to be a reality.

Ductal Cancer: Most breast cancers begin in the ducts that carry milk to the nipple for breastfeeding.

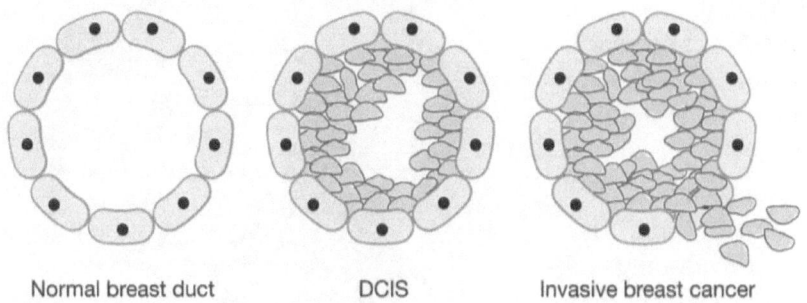

Normal breast duct   DCIS   Invasive breast cancer

Ductal In-Situ (DCIS) is stage 0 cancer located within a breast duct. It has not broken through the wall of the duct or spread into the surrounding breast tissue. Although not life threatening at this point, DCIS needs to be treated because there is the danger of it eventually becoming an invasive cancer. DCIS is usually picked up in a routine mammogram and successfully

11

treated with a lumpectomy (breast-conserving surgery) followed by radiation therapy.

Invasive ductal carcinoma (IDC) which is also known as infiltrating ductal carcinoma, is the most common form of breast cancer. It accounts for about 80 percent of all breast cancer diagnoses. IDC initially forms within a milk duct, breaks out of the duct wall, and spreads into the surrounding breast tissue. Left untreated, IDC has the potential to spread beyond the breast and travel to distant organs. IDC may be detected during a clinical breast exam, a mammogram, an MRI, and sometimes in a breast-self exam. Treatment may include one or more standard treatments such as surgery, radiation, chemotherapy, targeted therapy, and hormone therapy.

Lobular carcinoma in-situ (LCIS) describes the abnormal growth of cells in the lobules of the breast where milk is produced. While LCIS seldom progresses to an invasive cancer, lobular carcinoma in situ is considered a risk factor for developing a breast cancer in either breast. LCIS is most often found during a biopsy performed for another breast condition. Immediate treatment is not usually necessary, though following the condition closely is recommended. Women at high risk of developing a breast cancer may choose to have one or both breasts removed to lower 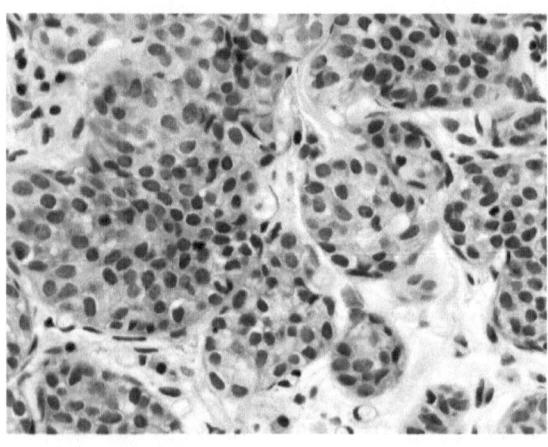 their chances of developing the disease.

Invasive lobular carcinoma (ILC), the second most common type of breast cancer, accounts for 8 percent of invasive breast cancers. ILC is less likely to present as a distinct lump. Treatment may include surgery, chemotherapy, radiation, and hormone therapy.

Inflammatory breast cancer (IBC) is an aggressive cancer, accounting for less than 5 percent of breast cancers. It usually does not present with a lump. IBC cancer cells infiltrate the breast skin and block its lymph vessels. Symptoms may include a rash and pitted skin. The affected breast may appear red, swollen and warm to the touch. It may initially be misdiagnosed as mastitis, an infection of the breast. Depending on the stage of the cancer at diagnosis, treatment may include surgery, chemotherapy, hormone treatment, and radiation treatment.

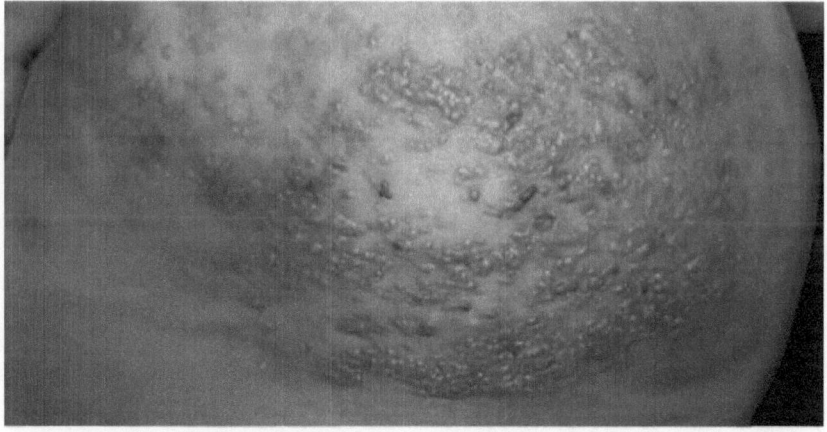

Paget's disease of the breast accounts for less than 3 percent of breast cancers. Symptoms may include nipple discharge, possible bleeding, and itchy, scaly skin similar to eczema, a skin condition. This breast cancer is usually diagnosed through performing a nipple biopsy. About 50 percent of patients with Paget's disease of the nipple have a tumor that can be felt in the breast during a clinical breast exam. Treatment will depend on the stage and other factors, including whether or not there is a cancerous tumor in the breast in addition to the Paget's disease.

Treatment may include surgery, chemotherapy, and hormone therapy.

Rare Types of Breast Cancer Include

Though it's less likely that you'll be diagnosed with one of these, if you're diagnosed at all, these rarer, lesser-known breast cancers are also worth being aware of.

Medullary carcinoma is considered a subtype of invasive ductal carcinoma. It has a spongy feel when touched; it does not feel like a lump. It can usually be seen on a mammogram. These tumors are rarely hormone receptor positive. Treatment options include surgery, radiation, and chemotherapy.

Tubular carcinoma is also considered a subtype of invasive ductal carcinoma. Its cells have a tubular appearance when looked at under a microscope. It feels spongy to the touch. It may be found during a clinical breast exam or a mammogram. Often not an aggressive cancer, it responds well to standard breast cancer treatments.

Mucinous carcinoma is considered a rare form of invasive ductal carcinoma cancer, in which the cells "float" in pools of mucin, a main ingredient of mucus. A diagnosis may take several steps, including a physical exam, a mammogram, ultrasound, an MRI, and a biopsy. Treatment, depending on the stage, may include surgery, chemotherapy, radiation, and hormone therapy.

Metastatic breast cancer is a stage IV breast cancer that has spread to other parts of the body, potentially including, but not limited to, the brain, bone, liver, and lungs. It is treatable, but unfortunately not curable. Less than 10 percent of those newly diagnosed with breast cancer have metastatic breast cancer when first diagnosed. Most metastatic breast cancers occur months or years after being diagnosed and treated for a localized breast cancer.

Treatment is ongoing, with the goals of providing not only quality, but length of life. In addition to possibly being treated with chemotherapy, radiation, and/or hormone therapy, women and men with metastatic breast cancer may opt to see if they qualify for participation in clinical trials of new treatments.

The Main Subtypes of Breast Cancer

Determining the subtype of a breast cancer is done during a biopsy, conducted by a pathologist, who is a medical doctor. The pathologist confirms the presence of cancer and further examines the tumor tissue looking for genetic and hormonal characteristics of the cancerous tumor.

The three main subtypes of breast cancer include:

Hormone-receptor-positive: Most breast cancer patients have this subtype of breast cancer; their tumors may be stimulated to grow and spread by either estrogen or progesterone. Hormone receptor positive tumors account for 65 to 75 percent of all tumors. It is treated with drugs such as tamoxifen, which can be taken by pre- and post-menopausal women, or aromatase inhibitors that can only be taken by patients who are post menopausal. The hormonal therapies block the activity of estrogen to reduce the chance of having a breast cancer recurrence.

HER2-positive: HER2 positive breast tumors (human epidermal growth factor 2), are "positive for a gene that codes for the HER receptor protein. While this receptor is necessary in the normal growth of breast cells, in excess (often 40 times to 100 times more common on these breast cancer cells than normal breast cells), the HER2 receptor may result in a cancer growing. Chemotherapy is the usual treatment.

Triple-negative: A triple-negative breast cancer does not have estrogen receptors, progesterone receptors, or HER2 receptors. Triple-negative tends to be more aggressive and affects almost 15 percent of those with breast cancer. Because triple-negative doesn't have hormone and HER2 receptors, it doesn't respond to hormone therapy, and chemotherapy is the recommended treatment.

Breast Cancer Clinical Presentation

History

Many early breast carcinomas are asymptomatic, particularly if they were discovered during a breast-screening program. Larger tumors may present as a painless mass. Pain or discomfort is not usually a symptom of breast cancer; only 5% of patients with a malignant mass present with breast pain.

Often, the purpose of the history is not diagnosis but risk assessment. A family history of breast cancer in a first-degree relative is the most widely recognized breast cancer risk factor.

The US Preventive Services Task Force (USPSTF) has updated its 2005 guidelines on risk assessment, genetic counseling, and genetic testing for BRCA-related cancer in women. The current USPSTF recommendations are as follows:

- Women who have family members with breast, ovarian, tubal, or peritoneal cancer should be screened to identify a family history that may be associated with an increased risk for mutations in the breast cancer susceptibility genes BRCA1 or BRCA2
- Women who have positive screening results should receive genetic counseling and then BRCA testing if warranted
- Women without a family history associated with an increased risk for mutations should not receive routine genetic counseling or BRCA testing

Physical Examination

If the patient has not noticed a lump, then signs and symptoms indicating the possible presence of breast cancer may include the following:

- Change in breast size or shape
- Skin dimpling or skin changes (e.g., thickening, swelling, or redness)
- Recent nipple inversion or skin change or other nipple abnormalities (e.g., ulceration, retraction, or spontaneous bloody discharge)
- Nipple discharge, particularly if blood stained
- Axillary lump

To detect subtle changes in breast contour and skin tethering, the examination must include an assessment of the breasts with the patient upright with arms raised. The following findings should raise concern:

- Lump or contour change
- Skin tethering
- Nipple inversion
- Dilated veins
- Ulceration
- Mammary Paget disease
- Edema or peau d'orange

The nature of palpable lumps is often difficult to determine clinically, but the following features should raise concern:

- Hardness
- Irregularity
- Focal nodularity
- Asymmetry with the other breast
- Fixation to skin or muscle (assess fixation to muscle by moving the lump in the line of the

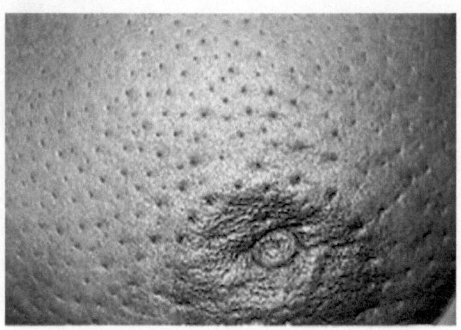

pectoral muscle fibers with the patient bracing her arms against her hips)

A complete examination includes assessment of the axillae and supraclavicular fossae, examination of the chest and sites of skeletal pain, and abdominal and neurologic examinations. The clinician should be alert to symptoms of metastatic spread, such as the following:

- Breathing difficulties
- Bone pain
- Symptoms of hypercalcemia
- Abdominal distention
- Jaundice
- Localizing neurologic signs
- Altered cognitive function
- Headache

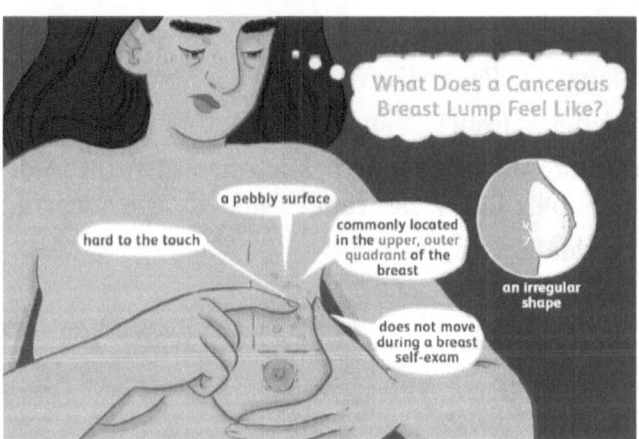

Workup

Approach Considerations

Breast cancer evaluation should be an ordered inquiry that begins with symptoms and a general clinical history. This is followed by a sequence that has become formalized as triple assessment, which includes the following components:

- Clinical examination
- Imaging (usually mammography, ultrasonography, or both)
- Needle biopsy

This approach naturally lends itself to a gradually increasing degree of invasiveness, so that a diagnosis can be obtained with the minimum degree of invasiveness and, consequently, the minimum amount of discomfort to the patient. Because the more invasive investigations also tend to be the most expensive, this approach is usually the most economical.

The aims of evaluation of a breast lesion are to judge whether surgery is required and, if so, to plan the most appropriate surgery. The ultimate goal of surgery is to achieve the most appropriate degree of breast conservation while minimizing the need for reoperation.

Breast cancer is often first detected as an abnormality on a mammogram before it is felt by the patient or healthcare provider. Mammographic features suggestive of malignancy include asymmetry, micro calcifications, and a mass or architectural distortion. If any of these features are identified, diagnostic mammography along with breast ultrasonography should be performed before a biopsy is obtained. In certain cases, breast magnetic resonance imaging (MRI) may be warranted.

Breast Cancer Screening

Whereas early detection has been advocated as a primary defense against the development of life-threatening breast cancer, questions have been raised in the past few years regarding the age at which to initiate, the modality to use, the interval between screenings, whether to screen older women, and even the impact on breast cancer related deaths. It is widely believed that breast tumors that are smaller or non-palpable and that present with a favorable tumor marker profile are more treatable when detected early.

A survival benefit of early detection with mammography screening has been demonstrated. A review that used seven statistical models determined that the use of screening mammography reduced the rate of death from breast cancer by 28–65% (median, 46%). A meta-analysis found that screening mammography reduces breast cancer mortality by about 20–35% in women 50–69 years old and slightly less in women 40–49 years old at 14 years of follow-up.

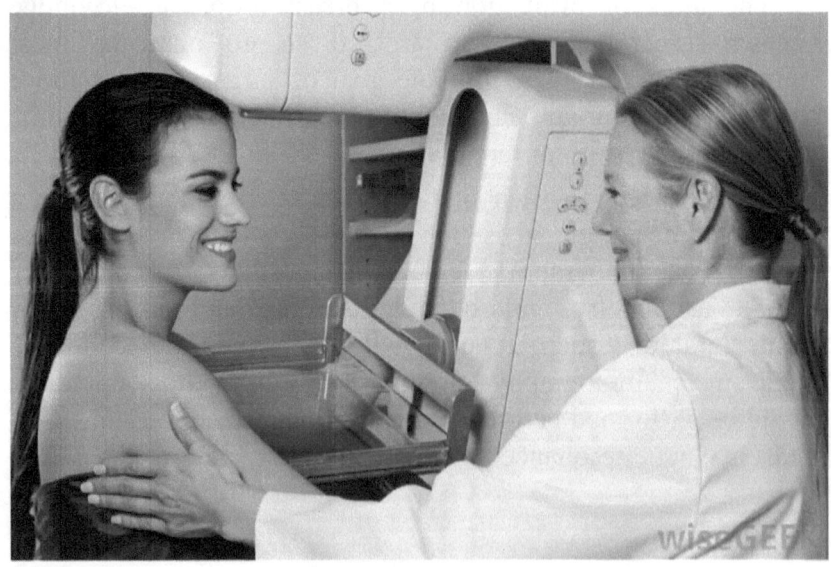

In the UK Age trial, breast cancer mortality in the first 10 years after diagnosis was significantly lower in women who received annual screening mammography from age 40-49 years than in those invited for screening at age 50 years and every 3 years thereafter. During the remainder of the 17-year follow-up period, however, reduction in breast cancer mortality was not evident.

In contrast, 25-year follow-up of 89,835 women in the Canadian National Breast Screening Study found that annual mammography in women aged 40-59 did not reduce mortality from breast cancer beyond that of physical examination or usual care when adjuvant therapy for breast cancer is freely available. Findings for women aged 40-49 and 50-59 were almost identical. Moreover, 22% (106/484) of invasive breast cancers detected by screening mammography were over-diagnosed, representing one over-diagnosed breast cancer for every 424 women who received mammography screening in the trial.

Mammogram

A mammogram is an x-ray of the breast. While screening mammograms are routinely administered to detect breast cancer in women who have no apparent symptoms, diagnostic mammograms are used after suspicious results on a screening mammogram or after some signs of breast cancer alert the physician to check the tissue.

Such signs may include:

- A lump
- Breast pain
- Nipple discharge
- Thickening of skin on the breast
- Changes in the size or shape of the breast

A diagnostic mammogram can help determine if these symptoms are indicative of the presence of cancer. As compared to screening mammograms, diagnostic mammograms provide a more detailed x-ray of the breast using specialized techniques. They are also used in special circumstances, such as for patients with breast implants.

What's Involved in A Diagnostic Mammogram?

If your doctor prescribes a diagnostic mammogram, realize that it will take longer than a normal screening mammogram, because more x-rays are taken, providing views of the breast from multiple vantage points. The radiologist administering the test may also zoom in on a specific area of the breast where there is a suspicion of an abnormality. This will give your doctor a better image of the tissue to arrive at an accurate diagnosis.

In addition to finding tumors that are too small to feel, mammograms may also spot ductal carcinoma in situ (DCIS). These are abnormal cells in the lining of a breast duct, which may become invasive cancer in some women.

How Reliable Are Mammograms For Detecting Cancerous Tumors?

The ability of a mammogram to detect breast cancer may depend on the size of the tumor, the density of the breast tissue, and the skill of the radiologist administering and reading the mammogram. Mammography is less likely to reveal breast tumors in women younger than 50 years than in older women. This may be because younger women have denser breast tissue that appears white on a mammogram. Likewise, a tumor appears white on a mammogram, making it hard to detect.

Ultrasound

When a suspicious site is detected in your breast through a breast self-exam or on a screening mammogram, your doctor may request an ultrasound of the breast tissue. A breast ultrasound is a scan that uses penetrating sound waves that do not affect or damage the tissue and cannot be heard by humans. The breast tissue deflects these waves causing echoes, which a computer uses to paint a picture of what's going on inside the breast tissue. A mass filled with liquid shows up differently than a solid mass.

The detailed picture generated by the ultrasound is called a "sonogram." Ultrasounds are helpful when a lump is large enough to be easily felt, and the images can be used to further evaluate the abnormality.

A breast ultrasound can provide evidence about whether the lump is a solid mass, a cyst filled with fluid, or a combination of the two. While cysts are typically not cancerous, a solid lump may be a cancerous tumor. Healthcare professionals also use this diagnostic method to help measure the exact size and location of the lump and get a closer look at the surrounding tissue.

MRI

During diagnostic examinations, it is helpful to get a variety of images and perspectives. If your initial exams are not conclusive, your doctor may recommend a breast MRI (magnetic resonance imaging) to assess the extent of the disease.

During a breast MRI, a magnet connected to a computer transmits magnetic energy and radio waves (not radiation) through the breast tissue. It scans the tissue, making detailed pictures of areas within the breast. These images help the medical team distinguish between normal and diseased tissue.

Positron Emission Tomography

Using a wide range of labeled metabolites (e.g., fluorinated glucose 18 FDG), positron emission tomography (PET) can detect changes in metabolic activity, vascularization, oxygen consumption, and tumor receptor status.

When PET is combined with computed tomography (CT) to assist in anatomic localization (PET-CT), scans can identify axillary and nonaxillary (e.g., internal mammary or supraclavicular) lymph node metastasis for the purposes of staging locally advanced and inflammatory breast cancer before initiation of neoadjuvant therapy and restaging high-risk patients for local or distant recurrences.

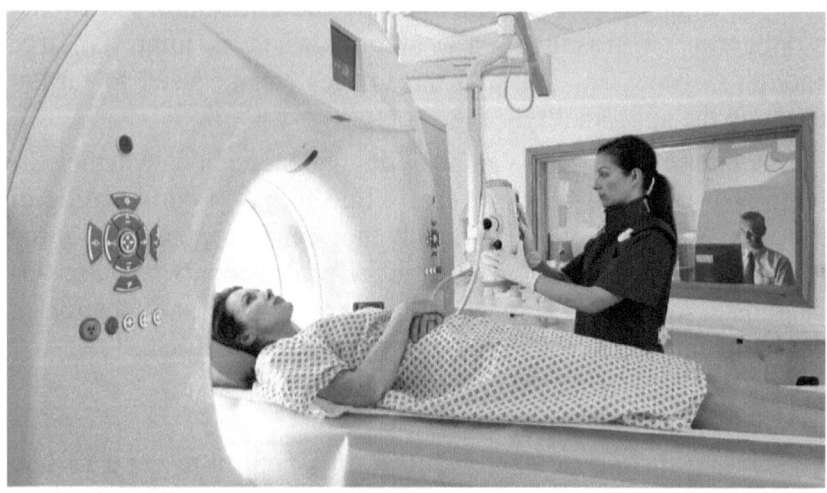

Scintimammography

Scintimammography is not indicated as a screening procedure for the detection of breast cancer. However, it may play a role in various specific clinical indications, as in cases of nondiagnostic or difficult mammography and in the evaluation of high-risk patients, tumor response to chemotherapy, and metastatic involvement of axillary lymph nodes.

In several prospective studies, overall sensitivity of scintimammography in the detection of breast cancer was 85%, specificity was 89%, and positive and negative predictive values were 89% and 84%, respectively.

Breast Biopsy

A breast biopsy is a test that removes tissue or sometimes fluid from the suspicious area. The removed cells are examined under a microscope and further tested to check for the presence of breast cancer. A biopsy is the only diagnostic procedure that can definitely determine if the suspicious area is cancerous.

The good news is that 80% of women who have a breast biopsy do not have breast cancer. There are three types of biopsies:

- Fine-needle aspiration
- Core-needle biopsy
- Surgical biopsy

The latter two are the most commonly used on the breast. There are several factors that help a doctor decide which type of biopsy to recommend. These include the appearance, size, and location of the suspicious area on the breast. Before discussing biopsy results, let's first distinguish between the three types of biopsies.

Fine-needle aspiration

In most cases, a fine needle aspiration is chosen when the lump is likely to be filled with fluid. If the lump is easily accessible or if the doctor suspects that it may be a fluid-filled cystic lump, the doctor may choose to conduct a fine-needle aspiration (FNA). During this procedure, the lump should collapse once the fluid inside has been drawn and discarded. Sometimes, an ultrasound is used to help your doctor guide the needle to the exact site, whereby sound waves create a picture of the inside of the breast.

If the lump persists, the surgeon or pathologist, will perform a fine needle aspiration biopsy (FNABx), a similar procedure using the needle to obtain cells from the lump for examination.

Core-needle biopsy

Core needle biopsy is the procedure to remove a small amount of suspicious tissue from the breast with a larger "core" (meaning "hollow") needle. It is usually performed while the patient is under local anesthesia, meaning the breast is numbed. During the procedure, the doctor may insert a very small marker inside the breast to mark the location of the biopsy. If surgery is later required, the marker makes it easier for the surgeon to locate the abnormal area.

The radiologist or surgeon performing the core-needle biopsy may use specialized imaging equipment to guide the needle to the desired site. As with fine-needle aspiration, this may involve ultrasound.

During an ultrasound-guided core needle biopsy, the patient lies down while the doctor holds the ultrasound against the breast to direct the needle. On the other hand, during a stereotactic-guided core-needle biopsy, the doctor uses x-ray equipment and a computer to guide the needle. Typically, the patient is positioned lying on the stomach on a special table that has an opening for the breast, and the breast is compressed, similar to a mammogram.

Occasionally, no imaging equipment is used, but this is typically only in cases where the lump can be felt through the skin. This type of procedure is called a freehand core-needle biopsy. There are fewer side effects associated with a core-needle biopsy than with surgical biopsy.

Surgical biopsy

It is also known as "wide local excision," "wide local surgical biopsy," "open biopsy," or "lumpectomy. As with a core-needle biopsy, a surgical biopsy is done while the patient is under local anesthesia. Typically, this test is performed in a hospital setting where an IV and medications are administered to make the patient drowsy.

The surgeon makes a one to two inch cut on the breast and then removes all or part of the abnormal lump and often a small amount of normal-looking tissue, known as the "margin." If the lump cannot be easily felt but can be seen on a mammogram or ultrasound, a radiologist may insert a thin wire to mark the suspicious spot prior to the surgeon performing the biopsy. Once again, a marker is usually placed internally at the biopsy site at the conclusion of the procedure.

Biopsy Results

Once the biopsy is complete, a specially trained doctor called a pathologist examines the tissue or fluid samples under a microscope, looking for abnormal or cancerous cells. The pathology report, which can take one or two weeks to complete, is sent to the patient's doctor. It indicates whether the suspicious area is cancerous and provides a full picture of your situation. For the patient, waiting for results can be a real challenge, but being able to make an informed decision regarding your treatment is well worth it. Your doctor will go over the report with you and, if necessary, discuss the treatment options.

If no cancer cells are found, the report will indicate that the cells in the lump are benign, meaning non-cancerous. However, some type of follow-up or treatment may still be needed, as recommended by the healthcare professional.

If cancer cells are found, the report will provide more information to help determine the next steps. The report for a core-needle biopsy sample will include tumor type and the tumor's growth rate or grade. If cancer is found, the pathologist will also perform lab tests to look at cells for estrogen or progesterone receptors.

In the case of a surgical biopsy, the results reveal data about the type, grade, and receptor status of the tumor, as well as the distance between the surrounding normal tissue and the excised tumor. The margin, as we mentioned earlier, shows whether the site is clear of cancer cells.

A positive margin means cancer cells are present at the margin of the tumor. In cases of positive margins, the cancer has spread beyond the immediate area. A negative margin or clear margin indicates there are no tumor cells at the margin. That means the cancer is contained in the area nearest to the tumor. A close margin means that the space between the cancerous tissue and surrounding normal tissue is less than about 3 millimeters.

If you have a biopsy resulting in a cancer diagnosis, the pathology report will help you and your doctor talk about the next steps. You will likely be referred to a breast cancer specialist, and you may need more scans, lab tests, or surgery. Your medical team uses the pathology report and the results of the other tests to determine the stage of cancer and to design the best treatment plan for you.

If you are diagnosed with breast cancer, your doctor may order additional lab tests to assist with prognosis. The two most common lab tests are the hormone receptor test and the HER2/neu test. Results from these tests can provide insight into which cancer treatment options may be most effective plan for you.

Lab tests for hormone receptors

A hormone receptor is a specialized protein located on the surface of or within a cell. The receptor binds to the female hormones estrogen and progesterone, which flow through the blood. Once bound, the hormone signals the cell to start growing and multiplying.

Many breast cancer tumors contain hormone receptors, often in large numbers. When hormone receptors are present, estrogen and/or progesterone can fuel the growth of the cancer. Such hormone-dependent cancers often respond well to hormone therapy, which differs from hormone replacement therapy (HRT). If neither estrogen receptors (ER) nor progesterone receptors (PR) are present, the cancer is said to be "hormone-receptor-negative," and hormone therapy would likely be ineffective. Knowing whether the cancer cells have hormone receptors can be valuable to your medical team and your treatment plan.

Who Needs Hormone Receptor Testing?

Hormone receptor testing is generally recommended for patients who are diagnosed with invasive breast cancer. If your doctor orders this test, you may be asked to discontinue taking any prescribed hormones for a period of time before the breast tissue sample is obtained. Usually, the sample comes from a biopsy, but the test may also be performed on tissue removed during a mastectomy.

How Does The Test Work?

The testing lab typically uses a specialized staining process on the breast tissue sample to see if hormone receptors are present. The technical name for this procedure is an "immunohistochemical staining assay" or an "ImmunoHistoChemistry (IHC)." Findings will be included in a pathology report given to your doctor. If the cancer is deemed "estrogen-receptor-positive" (ER+), its cells have receptors for the estrogen hormone. That means that the cancer cells likely receive signals from estrogen to promote growth. About two out of every three breast cancers contain hormone receptors.

If the cancer is progesterone-receptor-positive (PR+), its cells have receptors for the progesterone. This hormone could then promote the growth of the cancer.

What do the results of hormone testing mean?

Breast cancer patients who test positive for both estrogen receptors and progesterone receptors usually have a better-than-average prognosis for survival and a complete recovery than those who have no receptors present. Also, the more receptors and the more intense their reaction, the better they respond to hormone therapy. Patients with one type of receptor but not the other may still reap benefits from this form of treatment, but likely not to the same degree. As mentioned earlier, if the cancer is both ER- and PR-negative, it probably won't respond to hormone therapy. Typical response rates to hormone therapy are as follows:

- ER and PR positive: 75-80%
- ER positive and PR negative: 40-50%
- ER negative and PR positive: 25-30%
- ER negative and PR negative: 10% or less

HER2/neu Test

Similar to the hormone receptor test, the HER2/neu test looks for a specific kind of protein that is found with certain types of cancer cells and the gene that produces it. The formal name of that gene is the human epidermal growth factor receptor 2, and it makes HER2 proteins. These proteins are receptors on breast cells.

In a sense, genes contain the formula for the number and combination of proteins a cell needs to remain healthy and function properly. Certain genes and the proteins they create can determine how breast cancer progresses, as well as how it responds to various types of treatment.

What is a HER2 receptor and how does it relate to breast cancer?

Healthy HER2 receptors are the proteins that help manage how a breast cell grows, divides, and repairs itself. However, in about a quarter of all breast cancer patients, the HER2 gene isn't functioning properly. It makes an excess number of copies of itself in a process known as "HER2 gene amplification." Then these extra genes instruct the cells to make too many HER2 receptors, which is called "HER2 protein overexpression." The ultimate result is that breast cells grow and divide in an uncontrolled fashion.

The HER2/neu test can discover whether the sample is normal or whether it has too much of the HER2/neu protein or an excessive number of copies of its gene. If you have been diagnosed with invasive breast cancer or have had recurrent breast cancer, your doctor may recommend this test. It will help your medical team determine your prognosis, characteristics of the tumor including how aggressive the tumor is likely to be, and the best treatment options.

This test is often ordered in conjunction with the hormone receptor test. Typically, the breast cancer tissue sample from a biopsy or the tumor removed during a mastectomy is used.

What will the HER2/neu results tell me?

There are four tests for HER2, and results of these may appear on your pathology report, which may take several weeks to come back.

The first one is the IHC test, which is short for "ImmunoHistoChemistry." It looks at whether there is excess HER2 protein in the cancerous cells. A result of 0 or 1+ indicates there is no excess, 2+ is borderline, and 3+ means the cells test positive for HER2 protein overexpression.

The remaining three tests all examine if the cells contain too many copies of the HER2 gene. These tests include:

- **The FISH test** ("Fluorescence In Situ Hybridization")
- **The SPoT-Light HER2 CISH test** ("Subtraction Probe Technology Chromogenic In Situ Hybridization")
- **The Inform HER2 Dual ISH test** ("Inform Dual In Situ Hybridization")

There are only two possible results for these three tests: positive, meaning HER2 gene amplification, or negative, indicating the number of HER2 genes is not excessive.

In the pathology report, breast cancers with HER2 protein over expression and HER2 gene amplification are called HER2-positive. This type of cancer often grows faster, spreads to other areas more readily, and has a higher likelihood of recurring versus HER2-negative breast cancer.

Blood Testing for HER2/neu

Sometimes, especially when there is not enough tumor tissue available to perform the test, a blood sample is drawn from the patient's arm to collect similar data. This blood test is called a "serum HER2/neu test," and it can be used as part of the initial workup upon cancer diagnosis or to monitor the effectiveness of treatment. If initially the level of serum HER2/neu is elevated to more than 15ng/mL and then it falls, the treatment is likely working. However, if the serum level remains elevated, this indicates the treatment is not working. If the serum level declines but then, upon later testing, is elevated once again, this is a sign that the cancer could be recurring.

When all three of the tests come back negative for receptors for hormones (progesterone and estrogen) and negative for HER2, triple negative breast cancer may be the diagnosis.

Stages of breast cancer

Staging describes or classifies a cancer based on how much cancer there is in the body and where it is when first diagnosed. This is often called the extent of cancer. Information from tests is used to find out the size of the tumor, what part of the breast has cancer, whether the cancer has spread from where it first started and where the cancer has spread. Your healthcare team uses the stage to plan treatment and estimate the outcome (your prognosis).

The most common staging system for breast cancer is the TNM system. For breast cancer there are 5 stages – stage 0 followed by stages 1 to 4. Often the stages 1 to 4 are written as the Roman numerals I, II, III and IV. Generally, the higher the stage number, the more the cancer has spread. Talk to your doctor if you have questions about staging.

When describing the stage of breast cancer, sometimes doctors group them as follows:

In situ breast cancer – The cancer cells are only in the duct or lobule where they started and have not grown into nearby breast tissue (non-invasive). It is stage 0.

Early stage breast cancer – The tumor is smaller than 5 cm and the cancer has not spread to more than 3 lymph nodes. It includes stages 1A, 1B and 2A.

Locally advanced breast cancer – The tumor is larger than 5 cm. The cancer may have spread to the skin, the muscles of the chest wall or more than 3 lymph nodes. It includes stages 2B, 3A, 3B and 3C. Inflammatory breast cancer is also considered locally advanced breast cancer.

Metastatic breast cancer – The cancer has spread to other parts of the body. It is stage 4.

There are several groups of lymph nodes around each breast. The stage often depends on which lymph nodes the cancer has spread to.

Stage 0 (carcinoma in situ)

One of the following applies:

- There are cancer cells only in the lining of a breast duct. This is called ductal carcinoma in situ (DCIS).
- There is a buildup of abnormal cells in the breast lobules. This is called lobular carcinoma in situ (LCIS).
- There is Paget disease of the breast without any invasive carcinoma, DCIS or LCIS.

Stage 1A

The tumor is 2 cm or smaller.

Stage 1B

The tumor is 2 cm or smaller, or no tumor can be seen in the breast. A small number of cancer cells are found in the lymph nodes (micrometastases). Each lymph node with cancer cells in it is no larger than 2 mm.

Stage 2A

The tumor is 2 cm or smaller, or no tumor can be seen in the breast. Cancer cells are found in 1 to 3 lymph nodes under the arm (axillary lymph nodes), in lymph nodes inside the chest around the breastbone (internal mammary lymph nodes) or in both areas.

Or the tumour is larger than 2 cm but not more than 5 cm.

Stage 2B

The tumour is larger than 2 cm but not more than 5 cm. The cancer has also spread to 1 to 3 axillary lymph nodes, internal mammary lymph nodes or both areas.

Or the tumour is larger than 5 cm.

Stage 3A

The tumor is 5 cm or smaller, or no tumor can be seen in the breast. Cancer cells are found in 4 to 9 axillary lymph nodes, or in internal mammary lymph nodes but not in axillary lymph nodes.

Or the tumor is larger than 5 cm. The cancer has also spread to 1 to 9 axillary lymph nodes or to internal mammary lymph nodes. Or it may have spread to 1 to 3 axillary lymph nodes and internal mammary lymph nodes.

Stage 3B

The tumor has grown into the muscles of the chest wall or the skin or both. The cancer may have also spread to 1 to 9 axillary lymph nodes or to internal mammary lymph nodes. Or it may have spread to 1 to 3 axillary lymph nodes and internal mammary lymph nodes.

Or it is inflammatory breast cancer.

Stage 3C

It is stage 3C when any of the following applies:

- The cancer has spread to 10 or more axillary lymph nodes or to lymph nodes below the collarbone (infraclavicular lymph nodes).
- The cancer has spread to more than 3 axillary lymph nodes and internal mammary lymph nodes.
- The cancer has spread to lymph nodes above the collarbone (supraclavicular lymph nodes).

Stage 4

The cancer has spread to other parts of the body (called distant metastasis), such as to the bone, liver, lungs or brain. This is also called metastatic breast cancer.

Recurrent breast cancer

Recurrent breast cancer means that the cancer has come back after it has been treated. If it comes back in the same place that the cancer first started, it's called local recurrence. If it comes back in tissues or lymph nodes close to where it first started, it's called regional recurrence. It can also recur in another part of the body. This is called distant metastasis or distant recurrence.

Treatment

You've just been diagnosed with cancer. Your mind is reeling. And now your doctor wants you to sort through cancer treatment options and help decide on a plan. Naturally he will advise you surgery, chemotherapy and radiation, because that's what he has to offer you. He may show extreme urgency to start the treatment immediately. But there is no need to panic. Take your time. There are many safe and better alternative cancer treatments, which he doesn't know. You have to research and explore these wonderful therapies.

But how do you decide on a cancer treatment option? Here are five steps to guide you in determining right treatment for your cancer.

Step 1: Set your ground rules

- Before exploring treatment options, establish some ground rules. You'll be more comfortable with any cancer treatment decisions you make if you:

- Decide how much you want to know. While most people want to know exactly what their treatment is and their survival chances, others don't. If you don't want to know all the details, let your doctor or a relative know.

- Make sure you let your doctor know if you want someone else who might be able to help you during this difficult time to hear the news.

- Decide how you want to make your treatment decisions. You might want to take the lead in the decision-making process. Or you might want to turn all decisions over to your doctor or your spouse. You might also be somewhere in the middle, sharing the decision process with your doctor.

- It may help to think about how you've handled difficult decisions in the past. And it may help to have a close friend or family member at your appointments to help you decide.

- Have realistic expectations. Your doctor can give you estimates about what you can expect to get from each type of treatment. Exactly what side effects you may be willing to put up with will depend on what the benefits of the treatment are likely to be. Communicate your preferences with your doctor.

- Keep the focus on you. Don't let yourself be pressured into a particular treatment option. Pick what you feel most comfortable with.

- Accept help. You'll need support throughout your treatment. Support can come from your doctor, your friends and your family.

- It might help to write down your expectations and preferences before you meet with your doctor. That might help you better express your hopes for and feelings about your cancer treatment.

Step 2: Decide on a goal

- Deciding what you want out of treatment can help you narrow your treatment choices. Are you hoping for a cure, stabilization or solely symptom relief?

- Depending on your cancer type and stage, your goals for treatment might be:

  - **Cure** - When you're first diagnosed, it's likely you'll be interested in treatments that cure cancer. When a cure is possible, you may be willing to endure more short-term side effects in return for the chance at a cure.

  - **Control** - If your cancer is at a later stage or if previous treatments have been unsuccessful, you might adjust your goal to controlling your cancer. Different treatments may attempt to temporarily shrink or stop your cancer from growing. If this is your goal, you might not be willing to endure the side effects of harsher treatments.

- **Comfort** - If you have an advanced stage of cancer or one that hasn't responded to treatments, you might decide that comfort is most important to you. You and your doctor will work together to make sure you are free of pain and other symptoms.

Step 3: Research your treatment options

- To make a reasonable treatment decision, keep in mind the type of cancer you have, its stage, and what treatment options are available and how likely these treatments are to work under these circumstances. Talk to wise friend about trustworthy websites, books, alternative cancer therapies and patient education materials to supplement your discussions.

- Cancer treatments are sometimes used in conjunction with each other. For example, it's common to pair surgery or radiation with chemotherapy. Doctors sometimes refer to a treatment that's used after the primary treatment as an adjuvant therapy.

Step 4: Analyze the benefits versus the risks

Compare the benefits and risks of the different cancer treatments to decide which treatments fall within your goals. Rate the treatments you're considering based on the pros and cons of each. Some aspects you'll want to consider for each treatment include:

- **Side effects**. Take time to review the side effects of each treatment and decide whether they'll be worth enduring or too much to handle. Your doctor can give you a good idea of how common the various side effects are for each treatment and explain options for managing side effects to make treatment more tolerable.

- How treatment affects your life. Consider how treatment will affect your everyday life. Will you need a day off work or several weeks off? How will your role in your family change? Will you need to travel for your treatment? How will treatment affect your ability to find or keep employment? Understand that you have certain rights under the Americans with Disabilities Act, which covers patients with cancer and can help protect your employment.

- The financial costs of treatment. Investigate what types of treatment will be covered by your insurance. If a treatment or aspect of a treatment isn't covered, can you afford it? Call your insurance company to be sure.

- Your health in general. If you have other health conditions, ask your doctor how treatment will affect those conditions. For example, corticosteroids are commonly used in people with cancer. This could complicate diabetes treatment and affect your risk of cataracts, hypertension and osteoporosis.

- Your personal values and goals will make a difference in what treatments are best for you. Only you can decide what type of treatment will fit best in your life. But you don't have to make a choice and stick with it. It's very possible that you may change your mind during treatment, and that's fine.

Step 5: Communicate with your doctor

Effective communication with your doctor is the best way to make sure you're getting the information you need to make an informed decision. To make communicating with your doctor easier, try to:

- Speak up when you don't understand. If you need further explanation or clarification, tell your doctor. If you don't speak up, your doctor may think you understand.

- Write your questions in advance. Appointments can be stressful and emotional. Don't expect to remember all the questions you want to ask.

- Record your conversations. Try to keep track of what your doctor tells you by taking notes. You might also ask if it's OK to record the conversation. This record will be a good reference if you have questions later.

- Bring someone with you. If you feel comfortable sharing your medical information with a friend or family member, bring along someone to take notes. Then you'll have another person you can talk through your treatment decisions with.

- Keep copies of your medical records. Ask for copies of your medical records and bring them to each appointment.

- Don't expect you and your doctor to fully understand each other after one meeting. It may take a few conversations before you both feel as if you're on the same page.

Other things to keep in mind

As you're making your treatment decisions with your doctor, keep these points in mind:

- **Take your time**. Although a cancer diagnosis might make you feel as if you have to make immediate decisions to begin therapy, in most situations you have time to make choices. Ask your doctor how much time you have to decide.

- You can always change your mind. Making a treatment decision now doesn't bind you to that option. Tell your doctor if you're having second thoughts. Significant side effects may make you want to change your treatment plan.

- You can seek a second opinion. Don't be afraid of offending your doctor if you want to get a second opinion. Most doctors understand the need for a second opinion when facing a major decision.

- You don't have to be involved with treatment decisions. If you prefer, tell your doctor you'd rather not be involved in the decision-making process. You can always get involved later when you feel more comfortable with the situation. Let your doctor know who you want to make decisions about your care.

- You don't have to have treatment. Some people choose not to have treatment at all. People with very advanced cancers sometimes find they'd rather treat the pain and other side effects of their cancer so that they can make the best of the time they have remaining.

- If you choose not to be treated, you can always change your mind. Forgoing treatment doesn't mean you'll be left on your own, there are many ways of controlling side effects exist.

- Which treatment is best for you? There's no 100 percent right or wrong answer. But being involved with your treatment plan may give you greater peace of mind and can let you focus your energy on what you need to do most, keeping yourself healthy throughout your treatment.

Surgery

The first step and most common form of treatment for breast cancer is surgery. Surgery involves removing the tumor and nearby margins. The margin is the surrounding tissue that might be cancerous. The goal of surgery is to remove not only the tumor, but also enough of the margin to be able to test for the spread of the cancer. Once the removed tissue is checked, your post-operative report should tell you if you had "clear margins," (meaning the tissue farthest away from the breast was free of any cancer cells.)

Some people with Stage 2 or Stage 3 cancer may receive chemotherapy first, which is known as "pre-operative " or "neoadjuvant*" chemotherapy. The goal is to shrink the tumor.

By making it smaller first, you may have the option of a breast-conserving surgery or lumpectomy instead of a mastectomy.

*The term adjuvant means "helper" or "enhancer." Neo means "new" or "at the onset." So a neoadjuvant therapy is a helper therapy delivered at the beginning of treatment.

Either your doctor or a breast surgical oncologist (a breast surgeon specializing in breast cancer surgeries) will advise you regarding the surgery options to consider based on specific information about your breast cancer. You can discuss and compare the benefits and risks of each option and describe how well each possible choice can achieve the goal of ridding your body of the primary breast cancer.

Lumpectomy

A lumpectomy usually removes the least amount of breast tissue. The surgeon removes the cancer and a small portion or margin of the surrounding tissue, but not the breast itself. Even though the lumpectomy is the least invasive breast cancer surgery, it can still be very effective, and further surgery may not be needed.

Mastectomy

In the past, breast cancer surgery often required removing the entire breast, chest wall, and all axillary lymph nodes in a procedure called a radical mastectomy. While radical mastectomies are less common today, there are instances in which this surgery is the best option to treat the cancer.

If the cancer is detected early enough, there are usually options that will remove the cancer while preserving breast tissue. The common options are a lumpectomy (most often followed by breast radiation treatments) and a partial mastectomy.

Partial Mastectomy

A partial mastectomy requires the surgeon to remove a larger portion of the breast than in the lumpectomy — perhaps a whole segment or quadrant of tissue — in order to eliminate the cancer.

Occasionally, the surgeon will remove some of the lining over the chest muscles as well.

Skin-Sparing Mastectomy

This procedure requires removal of the breast, nipple, areola, and sentinel lymph node (or nodes) but not the breast skin. Many women who intend to have breast reconstruction will opt for this procedure.

Simple Mastectomy

This surgery requires removal of the breast, nipple, areola, and sentinel lymph node or nodes. It leaves the chest wall and more distant lymph nodes intact.

Coping With Change, Making Your Plan

After a mastectomy, you have several choices that can help you become comfortable with the changes in your body. They are all options with benefits to each approach. What is best for you and your body may not be what is best for another woman.

If you think you will opt for a breast reconstruction, you should speak with your medical team before you have the lumpectomy or mastectomy, even if you plan to wait until later to have your breast reconstruction.

Breast Reconstruction Options

There are a few options for breast reconstruction, and which one you use will depend on your age, body type, and treatment plan.

Breast Implants: The breasts are filled with sacs of saline or silicone gel.

Skin Grafts and Transplant: (TRAM Flap, Latissimus Flap, or Gluteal Flap)

An alternative solution is to use tissue the surgeon removes from another part of your body, like the belly (TRAM), back (latissimus), or buttocks (gluteal). The surgeon sculpts this tissue into the shape of your breast.

Additional Cosmetic Details: In addition to reconstructing the breast, the surgeon can add a nipple, change the shape or size of the reconstructed breast, and operate on the opposite breast as well for a better match. The plastic surgeon will be able to discuss with you the benefits and risks of each procedure and help you decide what will make you feel the most natural.

Are There Any Alternatives To Breast Reconstruction Surgery?

One alternative to breast reconstruction is a removable prosthetic breast that is worn in the bra. This will preserve the shape and look of the breast without the surgical procedures. Some women opt for prosthesis to help balance out their weight and posture, too.

Lymph Node Removal & Lymphedema

In addition to your surgical procedure, such as a lumpectomy or mastectomy, your doctor may wish to remove and examine lymph nodes to determine whether the cancer has spread and to what extent. Your doctor will use one of two procedures for this, either a sentinel lymph node biopsy/removal or an axillary node dissection. We'll define these terms below.

Although breast cancer is not easily controlled, the spread of breast cancer is sometimes predictable. The cancer cells spread through a customary path, out from the tumor and into the surrounding lymph nodes, before they progress throughout the body.

The sentinel lymph node (and in some cases there are several grouped together) is the first node "downstream" from the cancer in the lymph circulatory system. If the cancer were to travel away from the breast tumor and into the lymphatic system, this node would be the first one to show evidence of breast cancer.

Sentinel Node Biopsy

A sentinel lymph node biopsy is a procedure to examine the lymph node closest to the tumor because this is where the cancer cells have most likely spread. First, the surgeon will want to

45

identify the "sentinel lymph node," the lymph node (or nodes) closest to the tumor. To be able to identify the sentinel lymph node, the surgeon will inject dye or radioactive substances into the tissue near the tumor. The lymph nodes that are the most susceptible to the cancer's spread will be marked by the dye or radioactive substance. During surgery, the nearest lymph nodes will be removed and checked for the presence of cancer cells.

A biopsy is nearly always taken from the sentinel node, and the breast surgeon typically removes the sentinel node as well for dissection.

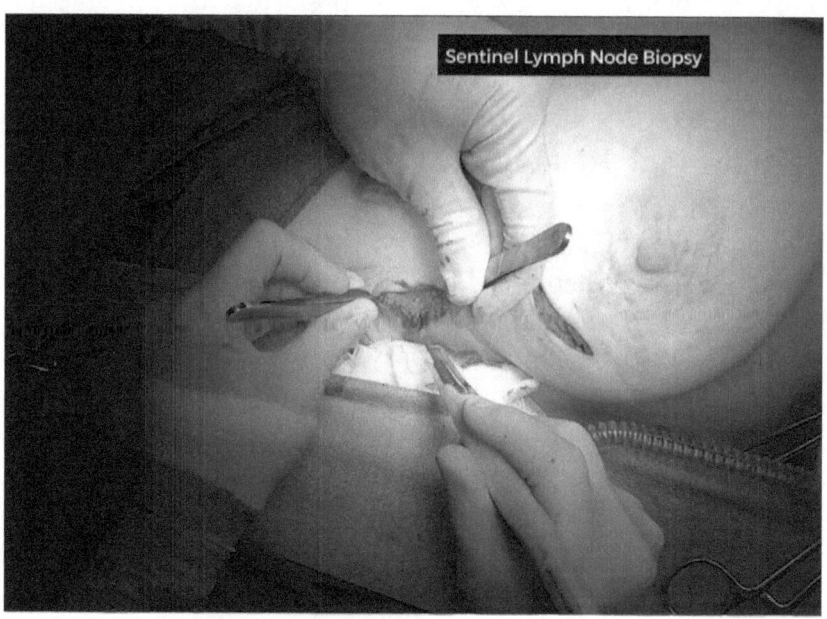

Axillary Node Dissection

This procedure is a method for determining if the cancer has spread to more than one of your lymph nodes. Axillary node dissection removes some of the axillary lymph nodes, which are the lymph nodes located in the underarm. Once removed, they are dissected and examined.

Do The Lymph Nodes Always Need To Be Removed?

Not always, especially when there is no evidence of any cancer in the lymph system. A mastectomy or lumpectomy operation will most often include either a sentinel node biopsy or an axillary node dissection. Both procedures involve a separate incision for lumpectomy patients. Following surgery, the pathologist will test the lymph nodes to determine whether the cancer has spread past the breast. When some evidence of cancer is found in the lymph system, recent standards are as follows:

For patients who are having a lumpectomy and the sentinel node is positive for cancer:

Effective in mid 2012, the standard of care was changed to no longer require women with early stage breast cancers to have a full dissection and removal of the lymph nodes under the arm. Instead radiation to the underarm can be planned.

For patients who are having a mastectomy surgery and have a positive sentinel node:

For these women, the standard of care remains the same, calling for the node removal and dissection of the axillary (or underarm) nodes. The additional nodes removed at the time of the breast cancer surgery will be examined by the pathologist in the following days to determine if others beyond the sentinel node contained cancer or not. If cancer cells are found in those lymph nodes, other cancer treatments will be considered.

What Is Lymphedema?

Lymphedema is a chronic condition that is caused by a disruption or damage to the normal drainage pattern in the lymph nodes. It most often causes swelling of the arm, but it can also affect the breast, chest, and sometimes even the legs. The swelling, caused by an abnormal collection of too much fluid, is called lymphedema. Removing the axillary lymph nodes increases your risk for developing lymphedema.

The risk of developing lymphedema continues for the rest of your life, so it is imperative that you are aware of these risks. Often it is best to learn about preventative measures for lymphedema before surgery so you will know the signs and symptoms to look for and can discuss treatment options with your physician.

After lymph node surgery, if you experience unusual and painful swelling, you should immediately notify your doctor to monitor it. It is very difficult to cure lymphedema, but your doctor can take steps to reduce swelling and maintain that reduction. With proper health care, good nutrition, and exercise, it may be possible for you to reduce the effects of lymphedema.

Modified Radical Mastectomy

This procedure requires removal of the entire breast, nipple, areola, and axillary lymph nodes but often leaves the chest wall intact.

Chemotherapy

Chemotherapy can be defined as the therapeutic use of chemicals to treat or control a disease. Chemotherapy for breast cancer is a systemic treatment, which affects most of the cells in your body. These toxic drugs are used to kill or delay the growth of cancer cells by disrupting their DNA, protein production, preventing cell division, starving them of nutrients, or blocking hormone receptors. Chemotherapy is commonly prescribed along with other treatment methods such as hormonal and targeted therapies. It can also be used to shrink a tumor before surgery for easier and safer removal.

Chemotherapy is offered to most patients based on several factors including:

- Tumor type
- Tumor grade
- Tumor size
- Type of receptors and status
- Number of lymph nodes involved and degree of involvement
- The risk for cancer to spread elsewhere in the body

Your medical team will work to select the right blend of chemotherapy drugs to suppress each stage of the cancer cells' growth.

How Are Chemotherapy Treatments Given?

Many chemotherapy drugs for breast cancer are given in a fluid form, as intravenous infusions, or injections, but are also available as pills or tablets. Some drugs may be given alone, and other drugs are combined to work together. When chemo drugs are given in combination, the treatment is called a regimen. Intravenous chemotherapy is given in infusions of 7- to 21-day cycles.

Typically, chemo is given once every three weeks, and you will need the intervening time to recover your blood counts and allow the drugs to work. Low-dose chemo is given weekly, as a smaller dose of drugs will require less recovery time. Oral chemo can be taken daily, or as directed. Injections may be given before, during, or after a chemo infusion.

Since chemotherapy drugs target fast-growing cells, your body will need time to rebuild healthy cells after each treatment. Most breast cancer chemo cycles are either once every three weeks for standard chemo or weekly for low-dose chemo.

Standard Chemo Schedule

Before each treatment, your medical oncologist may want you to take medications to protect against side effects. Be sure to take these on time as prescribed.

On the day of your infusion, plan on about four hours in the clinic. Your blood will be drawn and a complete blood count will be done. All your vital signs and weight will be taken, as that determines the amount of your dose of chemo drugs for that day.

Your oncologist will review your blood counts and if they are healthy enough, you will proceed to the infusion room for your chemotherapy treatment. If your blood counts are too low, further treatment may make you more vulnerable to infections or serious bleeding. Your chemotherapy will be delayed until your counts recover.

A Weekly Chemo Schedule

If you are receiving weekly lower-dose chemo, such as Taxol, you will receive a smaller dose than the typical dose given every three weeks. The smaller dose will usually be infused every week for 12 weeks straight. This will add up to more overall chemotherapy than you would receive on a standard schedule. You may also be given a white blood cell booster shot between infusion sessions.

The Day After Chemo

At least one day after each chemotherapy infusion, your blood will be drawn and counted. If there is concern that your red counts or neutrophils are low, you may be offered shots to boost those counts. Chemotherapy can greatly affect your blood counts because blood cells divide and multiply quickly.

Do not miss these extra appointments, so you can recover from chemo with a healthy immune system and avoid anemia and neutropenia.

Chemo Treatment Sequence

Here's how your chemotherapy appointments will be scheduled:

- Day Before: Take pre-chemotherapy medications (if prescribed) to prevent side effects.
- Day 1: Blood draw, weigh-in, vital signs, check-up, chemo infusion
- Day 2: Shots to boost blood counts if needed
- Day 3 and Until Next Cycle: Rest and recovery

Asking For Help Between Infusions

Between chemotherapy appointments, if you have trouble with side effects, don't hesitate to call your health care provider and ask for help. If you have become dehydrated after a treatment, you can ask for an infusion of saline fluid. Other medications may be given along with the saline, to help with nausea and vomiting.

Your chemotherapy nurses should know many tips for coping with side effects, so be sure to ask them for help, even if you don't have a scheduled appointment. Write down your symptoms—along with duration, severity, and how often they occur—before you call for help. This will help your nurses suggest ways to make you feel better.

Why Chemotherapy Causes Side Effects

The powerful nature of chemo treatment is both its strength and the reason behind its very bad reputation in regards to side effects. Chemo targets rapidly growing cells such as cancer. It may also affect your naturally fast-growing cells such as blood, mucous tissue in your digestive tract, finger and toenails, and hair follicles. These effects will subside after you've finished treatment.

How Can I Get Help Coping With Treatments?

Before each chemo infusion, you will be given medications to prevent nausea and vomiting. These may be pills, others may be fluids that are injected into your intravenous drip. After your infusion, you may need to take anti-nausea medications, so be

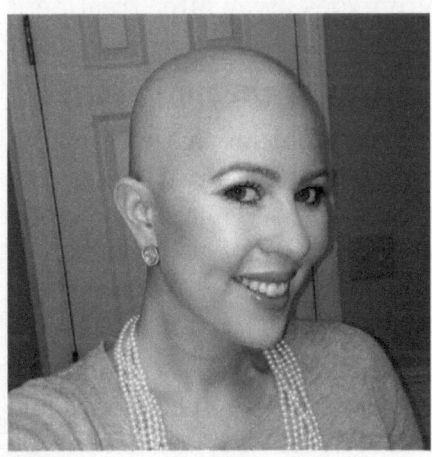

sure to get that prescription filled before your treatment. You may also be given anti-allergenic medications, or other substances to protect your healthy tissues. Be sure to let your doctor and nurses know what side effects you're having, and how severe those are. Ask for help managing the side effects. In most cases, the symptoms can be reduced or prevented.

What Are The Side Effects Of Chemotherapy?

Although chemotherapy kills the fast-growing cancer cells, the drugs can also unfortunately harm normal cells that divide rapidly.

You may have a reduction in red blood cells. When drugs lower the levels of healthy blood cells, you're more likely to get infections, bruise or bleed easily, and feel very weak and tired. Your healthcare team will check for low levels of blood cells. If your levels are low, your healthcare team may stop the chemotherapy for a while or reduce the dose of the drug. There are also medicines that can help your body make new blood cells.

Chemotherapy may affect the cells that produce hair. If you lose your hair, it will grow back after treatment, but the color and texture may be changed.

You may have changes from a different balance of cells lining your intestinal tract. Chemotherapy can cause a poor appetite, nausea and vomiting, diarrhea, or mouth and lip sores. Your healthcare team can prescribe medicines and suggest other ways to help with these problems.

Chemotherapy may affect the nerve cells. Some drugs used for breast cancer can cause tingling or numbness in the hands or feet. This problem often goes away after treatment is over.

Are there any lasting side effects of chemotherapy?

Sometimes people do experience problems that may not go away. For example, some of the drugs used for breast cancer may weaken the heart. Your doctor may check your heart before, during, and after treatment. A rare side effect of chemotherapy is that occasionally, years after treatment, a few women have developed leukemia (cancer of the blood cells).

Some anti-cancer drugs can damage the ovaries. If you have not gone through menopause yet, you may have hot flashes and vaginal dryness. Your menstrual periods may no longer be regular or they may stop. You may become infertile (unable to become pregnant).

Chemotherapy Affects Your Present and Future Fertility

If you are premenopausal before starting treatment, be aware that chemo can put you into temporary or permanent menopause. Your periods may stop, and you could experience medical menopause, which may be temporary or permanent. Specific chemo drugs are known to cause infertility.

If you have any thoughts about future pregnancies, let your oncologist know before you start treatment. Ask what your options are if you're planning to add to your family. Depending on your age, drug regimen, and dosage, your fertility may return after treatment. But if there is a chance that you will become infertile, you need to know before your first chemo infusion.

Chemotherapy Medicines

Chemotherapy medications for breast cancer include:

- Abraxane (chemical name: albumin-bound or nab-paclitaxel)
- Adriamycin (chemical name: doxorubicin)
- Carboplatin (brand name: Paraplatin)
- Cytoxan (chemical name: cyclophosphamide)
- Daunorubicin (brand names: Cerubidine, DaunoXome)
- Doxil (chemical name: doxorubicin)
- Ellence (chemical name: epirubicin)
- Fluorouracil (also called 5-fluorouracil or 5-FU; brand name: Adrucil)
- Gemzar (chemical name: gemcitabine)
- Halaven (chemical name: eribulin)
- Ixempra (chemical name: ixabepilone)
- Methotrexate (brand names: Amethopterin, Mexate, Folex)

- Mitomycin (chemical name: mutamycin)
- Mitoxantrone (brand name: Novantrone)
- Navelbine (chemical name: vinorelbine)
- Taxol (chemical name: paclitaxel)
- Taxotere (chemical name: docetaxel)
- Thiotepa (brand name: Thioplex)
- Vincristine (brand names: Oncovin, Vincasar PES, Vincrex)
- Xeloda (chemical name: capecitabine)

In many cases, chemotherapy medicines are given in combination, which means you get two or three different medicines at the same time. These combinations are known as chemotherapy regimens. In early stage breast cancer, standard chemotherapy regimens lower the risk of the cancer coming back. In advanced breast cancer, chemotherapy regimens make the cancer shrink or disappear in about 30-60% of people treated. Keep in mind that every cancer responds differently to chemotherapy.

Standard chemotherapy regimens include:

- **AT**: Adriamycin and Taxotere
- **AC ± T**: Adriamycin and Cytoxan, with or without Taxol or Taxotere
- **CMF**: Cytoxan, methotrexate, and fluorouracil
- **CEF**: Cytoxan, Ellence, and fluorouracil
- **FAC**: fluorouracil, Adriamycin, and Cytoxan
- **CAF**: Cytoxan, Adriamycin, and fluorouracil
- **TAC**: Taxotere, Adriamycin, and Cytoxan
- **GET**: Gemzar, Ellence, and Taxol

(The FAC and CAF regimens use the same medicines but use different doses and frequencies)

Depending on the characteristics of the cancer, a targeted therapy medicine, such as Herceptin (chemical name:

trastuzumab), may be used in combination with some chemotherapy regimens. For example, the TCH regimen includes Taxotere, Herceptin, and carboplatin.

Your doctor may talk about certain groups of chemotherapy medicines:

Anthracyclines are chemically similar to an antibiotic. Anthracyclines damage the genetic material of cancer cells, which makes the cells die. Adriamycin, Ellence, and daunorubicin are anthracyclines.

Taxanes interfere with the way cancer cells divide. Taxol, Taxotere, and Abraxane are taxanes.

Most standard chemotherapy regimens include a medicine from one or both of these groups.

Radiation Therapy

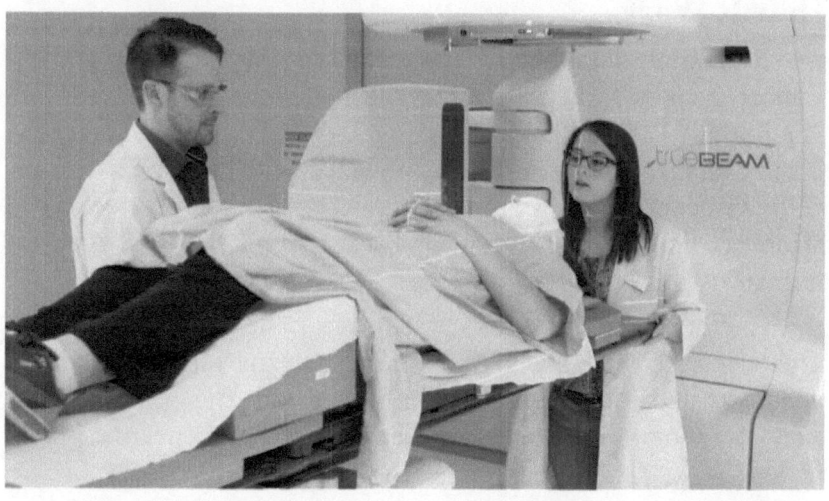

Radiation therapy, also known as radiotherapy, is sometimes used to treat breast cancer. It involves the use of ionizing radiation to kill cancer cells, either for curative purposes if a tumor is localized or palliative care to ensure comfort and quality of life if a malignancy cannot be cured. It can also be used in adjuvant therapy to prevent cancer recurrence after the tumor has been removed in a lumpectomy or mastectomy.

Not all women with breast cancer need radiation therapy. It is generally indicated in the following circumstances:

- After breast-conserving surgery to kill all remaining malignant cells so that the cancer does not return
- After a mastectomy if the tumor is larger than 5 centimeters (roughly two inches) or if nearby lymph nodes have evidence of cancer
- With stage 4 breast cancer when the cancer has spread (metastasized) from the breast to other organs in the body

Broadly speaking, there are two types of radiation therapy used to treat breast cancer: external beam radiation and brachytherapy (also known as internal radiation therapy). Each has its specific purpose and indications.

How It Works

Radiation is applied to cancer cells to impede their growth. Cancer cells are different from normal cells in that they are "immortal." Rather than undergoing apoptosis (programmed cells death) so that old cells can be replaced with new ones, cancer cells will continue to multiply unimpeded. Moreover, they do so at an accelerated rate, allowing them to infiltrate and supplant normal tissues.

Radiation therapy works by damaging the genetic material of a cancer cell, called DNA. By doing so, the radiation induces apoptosis and effectively kill the cancer cell. Beyond the tumor site, radiation can be used to clear cancer from nearby lymph nodes.

To minimize damage to nearby tissues, the affected area will first be mapped using a 3D imaging study, typically computed tomography (CT). This not only includes the tumor site but surrounding tissues, called margins, where cancer cells comingle with normal ones.

Once mapped, the tumor site can be irradiated from different angles either externally (with ionizing radiation beams) or internally (with encapsulated radioactive materials). Newer techniques are being developed that combine real-time imaging with the actual radiation procedure.

External Beam Radiation

External beam radiation is the most common form of radiation therapy used in breast cancer. The radiation is delivered by a machine that emits a single beam of high-intensity X-ray from several directions. The procedure is painless and relatively fast but can cause side effects.

The areas of irradiation can vary by whether you have had a mastectomy or lumpectomy and whether nearby lymph nodes are affected. The guidelines for external beam radiation can be broadly described as follows;

- If you have had a mastectomy and no lymph nodes are involved, radiation would be focused on the chest wall, the mastectomy scar, and the tissues were surgical drains were placed.

- If you had a lumpectomy, the entire breast would likely be irradiated (referred to as whole breast radiation) with an extra boost of radiation to the area where the tumor was removed (called the tumor bed).

- If axillary lymph nodes are involved, radiation may be delivered in the armpit and, in some cases, to the supraclavicular lymph nodes above the collarbone and the internal mammary lymph nodes in the center of the chest.

Radiation can also be used with chemotherapy if a tumor cannot be surgically removed. In cases of inflammatory breast cancer, an aggressive form that spreads through lymph channels in the breast, radiation may be used after breast surgery and chemotherapy.

Procedure

External beam radiation treatments would not start until you have healed from breast surgery or completed chemotherapy. The entire schedule of radiation therapy (called the course) is divided into daily treatments (referred to as fractions).

Before radiation therapy begins, a radiologist will map the treatment area and, along with the radiation oncologist and possibly a dosimetrist, determine the correct dose and angles of irradiation. The oncologist may apply small ink marks or tattoos to your skin to ensure the radiation is focused correctly.

(Speak with your oncologist in advance of the procedure to determine which, if any, ink marks will be permanent.)

The traditional schedule of whole breast radiation is five days a week, Monday through Friday, for five to six weeks. Each session lasts between 15 and 30 minutes.

In some cases, accelerated breast irradiation (ABI) may be used in which stronger radiation doses are given over a shorter period of time. There are several types of ABI used when appropriate:

- Hypofractionated radiation therapy is used in women who have undergone a lumpectomy and have no evidence of lymph node involvement. While the procedure is similar to conventional external beam radiation, the dose is higher and the treatment course is reduced to three weeks.

- 3D-conformal radiotherapy involves a specialized machine that only treats the immediate tumor site rather than the whole breast. It is typically used after a lumpectomy in women with no lymph node involvement. Treatment is delivered twice daily for five days.

- Intraoperative radiation therapy (IORT) also involves specialized equipment and is intended for women with early-stage cancer and no lymph node involvement. For this procedure, a single large dose of radiation is delivered immediately after the lumpectomy while the incision is still open.

Side Effects

Because the external beam radiation is delivered through the skin, it can "spill over" and affect other tissues, including the lungs, ribcage, and surrounding muscles. It can cause both short- and long-term side effects, depending on the size of the dose, the duration of therapy, the location of the tumor, and your general health. Common short-term side effects include:

- Fatigue
- Breast swelling
- Skin changes (including redness, darkening, or peeling)

These side effects typically resolve once the therapy is completed. Some may take longer to improve than others. Skin changes especially can take up to a year to normalize and, even then, may not fully return to its pretreatment state.

Long-term side effects may also occur due to the accumulative exposure to radiation. These include:

- Radiation-induced fibrosis (the hardening of breast tissue, often accompanied by decreased breast size and difficulty breastfeeding)
- Brachial plexopathy (localized nerve damage resulting in arm numbness, pain, and weakness)
- Lymphedema (lymph gland obstruction characterized by a swollen arm and surrounding tissues)
- Radiation-induced osteopenia (localized bone loss resulting in an increased risk of rib fracture)
- Angiosarcoma (a rare complication in which radiation therapy triggers cancer)
- In the past, external beam radiation posed a significant risk of heart and lung damage. Newer generation machines have largely alleviated the risk by reducing radiation spill-over.

Brachytherapy

Brachytherapy, also known as internal radiation therapy, is used after a lumpectomy to irradiate the surgical cavity from within. The radiation is delivered through one or several tubes, called catheters that are inserted through the skin of the breast. Radioactive seeds, pellets, tapes, or ribbons are then fed into the catheters and left for several minutes or days before being removed.

- Brachytherapy can be used with whole breast radiation or on its own as a form of accelerated partial breast irradiation (APBI). There are two types of brachytherapy commonly used in breast cancer:
- Interstitial breast brachytherapy involves the placement of several catheters in the breast through which radiation sources are strategically placed in and around the tumor site.
- Intracavity breast brachytherapy, also known as balloon brachytherapy, is used after a lumpectomy to deliver radiation to the breast cavity via an inflatable balloon filled with radioactive pellets.

Another type of brachytherapy, known as permanent breast seed implant (PBSI), may be used in early-stage cancer. It involves the permanent implantation of low-dose radioactive seeds to prevent cancer recurrence. After a week or so, the seeds will lose their radioactivity and begin to deteriorate.

Procedure

As with external beam radiation, brachytherapy requires the careful mapping of the surgical cavity. Prior to the delivery of radiation, one or more catheters would be inserted into the breast either during the lumpectomy or in a separate procedure. The catheters would be kept in place for the duration of therapy with a short length of tubing extending outside of the breast.

The type and dose of radioactive materials (typically iodine, palladium, cesium, or iridium) can vary by the treatment approach. They can range from ultra-low-dose rate (ULDR) seeds used for PBST to high-dose-rate (HDR) implants commonly used for APBI.

Once the correct dose and coordinates have been established, the external catheter would be connected to a machine, called an after loader, which feeds the radioactive source through the catheters and removes them once the fraction is complete.

Compared to the five to six weeks needed for external beam radiation, breast brachytherapy can be completed in anywhere from three or seven days.

Intracavity brachytherapy is commonly performed over five days and involves two 10- to 20-minute sessions delivered six hours apart. Interstitial brachytherapy, less commonly used today, may be performed as an in-hospital procedure over one or two days.

Side Effects

Brachytherapy can cause many of the same side effects of external beam radiation, although they tend to be less severe.

Because brachytherapy involves one or more small incisions, there is an added risk of infection (particularly if the catheter site is not cleaned or is allowed to get wet). In some cases, a pocket of fluid, called a seroma, may develop beneath the skin and require drainage with a syringe and needle.

Proton Beam Therapy

Proton beam therapy, also known as proton therapy, is an advanced method of radiation that poses less harm to surrounding tissues. Unlike high-intensity X-ray, which scatters radiation as it passes through a tumor, the radiation emitted in proton therapy does not travel beyond the tumor.

Instead, the charged particles, called protons, only release their energy as they reach their target. This reduces the so-called "exit dose" of radiation that can harm collateral tissues. Side effects are similar to other types of radiation therapy but are presumed to be less severe.

Although proton therapy has been around since 1989 and is already used to certain cancers (including prostate cancer and lymphoma), research is ongoing as to whether it would be effective for treating breast cancer.

Most of the current studies are focused on its use in early-stage and advanced localized breast cancer.

Beyond the absence of clinical research, the cost and availability of proton remain significant barriers to use. To date, there are only 27 centers equipped with proton beam cyclotrons in the United States, while the cost of treatment is generally two to three times that of external beam radiation.

Hormone Therapy

Hormonal therapies are often the first step in treating metastatic breast cancer, at least for those who have tumors which are estrogen receptor positive. The choice of medications will depend on whether you are premenopausal or postmenopausal, as well as if your cancer recurred while you were using one of these medications. (If your cancer recurred while taking one of these drugs it's thought that your cancer is likely resistant to the drug.)

Role of Estrogen

For estrogen receptor-positive breast cancers, estrogen works like fuel, binding with estrogen receptors on the surface of cancer cells and stimulating the growth and proliferation of cancer. This action of estrogen on cancer cells can be limited in a few different ways; by decreasing the amount of estrogen in the body, or by blocking estrogen receptors so estrogen is unable to stimulate the growth of the cells. In contrast to chemotherapy drugs which kill cancer cells directly (simplistically), hormonal therapies work by essentially "starving" the cancer cells of estrogen.

Prior to menopause, your ovaries are the biggest producers of estrogen. After menopause, the greatest source of estrogen in the body is from the conversion of androgens to estrogen. This conversion is catalyzed by the enzyme aromatase found in fat and muscle. Aromatase inhibitors are medications which block aromatase so that this conversion of androgens to estrogens cannot occur, effectively lowering estrogen levels.

Hormonal therapies are not effective for those who have estrogen receptor and progesterone receptor negative tumors.

It's also important to note that some estrogen receptor-positive tumors are also HER 2 positive. In tumors that are positive for both of these receptors, anti-estrogen therapy may be used with or without drugs which act on HER 2.

Premenopausal Therapy

If you are premenopausal, your ovaries are still the largest source of estrogen, and hence the fuel, for breast cancer. The goal of treatment in premenopausal women is thus to reduce the ability of estrogen to stimulate the growth of your cancer by either decreasing the amount of estrogen available (ovarian suppression therapy) and interfering with the ability of estrogen to bind with estrogen receptors on breast cancer cells.

Medications such as tamoxifen are referred to as SERMS—selective estrogen receptor modulating agents, and work by binding to cancer cells so that estrogen present in the body is unable to bind to the cell and signal the cell to grow.

It's thought that aromatase inhibitors may be more effective than tamoxifen, but these cannot be used in premenopausal women due to the activity of the ovaries. To reduce the estrogen produced by the ovaries, and allow you to use an aromatase inhibitor, your oncologist may recommend ovarian suppression therapy.

Ovarian suppression may be accomplished by:

- Using the medication **Zoladex (goserelin)** – This is a medication given subcutaneously and suppresses the production of estrogen by the body, and is known as a gonadotropic releasing hormone antagonist. The ovaries produce estrogen in response to a hormone known as gonadotropin stimulating hormone secreted by the pituitary gland. Zoladex inhibits the ability of the gonadotropin stimulating hormone to stimulate the ovaries.

- **Oophorectomy** – Less commonly, some women choose to have their ovaries removed (through a procedure called an oophorectomy) rather than using Zoladex. This surgery is done less often due to the greater risks associated with surgery, but some women may prefer this method, especially those who have a predisposition to ovarian cancer as well as breast cancer.

- An oophorectomy can often be done as a laparoscopic procedure and is usually the same day surgery. In a laparoscopic oophorectomy, a few small incisions are made in the abdomen and the ovaries are removed with the assistance of special instruments.

Following ovarian suppression therapy, premenopausal women can then be treated with medications as for postmenopausal women discussed below or with tamoxifen.

Postmenopausal Therapy

After menopause, the largest source of estrogen in the body comes from the peripheral conversion of androgen to estrogen. Postmenopausal breast cancer may be treated with tamoxifen (to block this peripherally converted estrogen from binding with cancer cells) but the category of medications called aromatase inhibitors appear to be more effective with fewer side effects.

Available aromatase inhibitors include:

- **Arimidex** (anastrozole)
- **Femara** (letrozole)
- **Aromasin** (exemestane)

Aromatase inhibitors may be used alone, or in combination with a chemotherapy medication. For example, the combination of Femara (letrozole) and Ibrance (palbociclib) and Aromasin (exemestane) with Afinitor (everolimus). There is always a balance when adding another medication. While the combination may be more effective, there is also an increase in side effects when combining more than one medication.

It's helpful to note again that the goal of treatment is often different with metastatic breast cancer than it is with early-stage breast cancer. With early stage breast cancer, the goal is curative, and the philosophy is to "pull out the big guns" to potentially cure the disease. The philosophy with metastatic breast cancer, in contrast, is often to control the growth of cancer with the least amount of medication possible, saving other medications for a time when the first medications no longer work.

Other Hormonal Treatments

In addition to tamoxifen and aromatase inhibitors, there are a few other hormone-related medications that may be used for metastatic breast cancer. If a breast cancer continues to grow or spread on the above medications it is usually considered resistant to these medications. Metastatic breast cancer almost always becomes resistant to these medications over time. When this happens, options include:

- **Faslodex (fulvestrant)** - For postmenopausal women who have progression of their cancer on tamoxifen or an aromatase inhibitor, an option is using the medication Faslodex. Faslodex is currently the only medication approved for breast cancer in a category known as SERD's—selective estrogen receptor down regulators.

This medication is referred to as a "pure antiestrogen" and blocks the effect of estrogen on estrogen receptor-positive breast cancer cells but in a different way than tamoxifen (it is an estrogen receptor antagonist.) Faslodex may be used alone or in combination with Ibrance (palbociclib), a chemotherapy drug, and given as an injection.

Infrequently Used Medications

There are other hormonal therapies which are used infrequently but are sometimes considered as a 3rd line or 4th line treatment. These include:

- **Fareston (toremifene)** – Fareston is a medication similar to tamoxifen and also considered an estrogen receptor modulating agent may sometimes be considered for postmenopausal women with estrogen receptor-positive breast cancers, particularly for women who lack an enzyme that converts tamoxifen to its active form in the body.

- **Progestins** - Megace (megestrol) is a synthetic form of progesterone that is sometimes used for people with estrogen receptor-positive breast cancer which has become resistant to tamoxifen. It was used more frequently in the past before newer drugs became available.

- **Sex steroid hormones** – Hormones such as estrogen and androgens are not commonly used with metastatic breast cancer, but may sometimes be used when other hormone treatments have failed.

Therapies for Men

Men with metastatic breast cancer which is hormone receptor positive are usually treated with tamoxifen.

Side Effects

Tamoxifen

Tamoxifen has different functions, both mimicking the effect of estrogen in some parts of the body and counteracting it in others. The most common symptoms include hot flashes and body aches which have been coined "old lady syndrome" though these body aches are often milder than with aromatase inhibitors.

Serious side effects include an increased risk of blood clots in the legs (venous thromboembolism) which, if untreated, have the potential to break free and travel to the lungs (pulmonary emboli.) Over time, tamoxifen may also cause uterine bleeding and is associated with a small increase in the development of uterine cancer.

Some women (and men) taking tamoxifen may develop a worsening of their symptoms (for example, increased redness of skin metastases or increased bone pain from bone metastases) within a few days of starting the medication.

If you develop these symptoms, they will usually resolve within four to six weeks, though sometimes the medication needs to be discontinued. The silver lining if you have this reaction is that a flare reaction is considered a sign that the medication is working and will be effective. Zoladex may also cause a similar flare reaction.

Note that Tamoxifen may cause abnormal liver function tests, anemia, and low platelets and is associated with an increased risk of endometrial cancer. Discuss with your doctor if this option is best for you.

Aromatase inhibitors (AI's)

AI's can also cause body aches, with around 40 percent of people noting some degree of muscles and joint aching. Bone loss is a side effect, and your oncologist will likely order a bone density to check you for osteoporosis, both at the beginning of treatment and periodically thereafter. Fractures may occur due to the bone loss, even without bone metastases. AI's may also increase the risk of heart disease.

Faslodex

Faslodex is usually fairly well tolerated, with the most common side effects being hot flashes and elevations of liver function tests.

Zoladex (goserelin)

One of the more common side effects of this medication is actually the effect that is desired. The goal of treatment is to suppress the ovaries, in other words, stop the ovaries from releasing estrogen. In doing this it essentially causes a medically induced menopause and thus, the normal symptoms of menopause such as hot flashes and vaginal dryness are common.

As with tamoxifen, some people may have a flare reaction when first starting the medication, for example, an increase in bone pain in those with bone metastases.

Oophorectomy

The primary side effects related to removing the ovaries are, as with medical hormone suppression therapy, the normal symptoms common with menopause such as hot flashes and vaginal dryness. There are also the side effects and risk related to surgery. An oophorectomy can now be done with minimally invasive surgery (a laparoscopy) through a few small cuts in the skin and is usually done as a same-day surgical procedure.

Faslodex (fulvestrant)

Since this is an anti-estrogen medication, most of the symptoms are similar to those found with menopause, like with tamoxifen and the aromatase inhibitors. Roughly a third of people experience mild nausea, but otherwise, this medication is usually well tolerated.

Targeted Therapy

Targeted therapies are a relatively new form of treatment for breast cancer and may be used alone or in combination with other treatments. Unlike traditional chemotherapy which attacks any rapidly growing cells, targeted therapies directly target cancer cells or signaling pathways which contribute to the growth of cancer cells. For this reason, many of the drugs may have fewer side effects than chemotherapy.

Targeted therapies are available for those with estrogen receptor-positive breast cancers, HER 2 positive breast cancers, and even triple negative breast cancer.

These drugs can work very well, but like the other medications used to treat metastatic breast cancer, resistance usually develops over time. Some of these drugs are used for both early stage and metastatic breast cancer, whereas others are used primarily for people with metastatic breast cancer.

Therapies for HER2 Positive Cancer

In around 25 percent of breast cancers, a gene known as human epidermal growth receptor 2 (or HER 2/neu) results in the overexpression of the HER 2 protein (receptors) on the surface of breast cancer cells.

Similar to the mechanism by which estrogen receptors are responsible for signaling a cancer cell to grow and proliferate, HER 2 receptors may result in the growth and proliferation of HER 2 positive cancers. Medications that interfere with these receptors thus interfere with the signal to these cancer cells, limiting their growth.

Medications that target HER 2 include:

- **Herceptin (trastuzumab):** Herceptin, one in a class of drugs called monoclonal antibodies, is given intravenously (IV), usually once a week or once every three weeks. Side effects include fever and chills early on. Heart failure may develop in 3 percent to 5 percent of people treated with the drug, but unlike the heart failure related to chemotherapy drugs such as Adriamycin (doxorubicin), this heart failure may be reversible when the treatment is stopped. Side effects from Herceptin usually improve over time.

- **Kadcyla (ado-trastuzumab):** Kaydcyla is a medication which includes both Herceptin and a very potent chemotherapy drug called emtansine. The Herceptin portion of the drug binds to HER 2 positive cancer cells, but instead of simply blocking the receptor to prevent growth hormones from attaching, Herceptin allows the chemotherapy to enter the cancer cells, where the emtansine is released. While this chemotherapy agent is mostly delivered right to cancer cells, there is also some general absorption of the drug into the system. For this reason, the drug may have side effects common to chemotherapy drugs, including bone marrow suppression and peripheral neuropathy. Kaydcla may be effective even in people for whom Herceptin has been ineffective.

- **Perjeta (pertuzumab):** Perjeta, a monoclonal antibody, was FDA-approved for metastatic breast cancer in 2013 and studies have subsequently found an increase in the survival rate for women with metastatic breast cancer (HER 2 positive) who are treated with the drug. It may be used alone or in combination with Herceptin or chemotherapy.

- **Tykerb (lapatinib):** Tykerb also attacks HER 2 positive breast cancer cells, but by a different mechanism than Herceptin. Tykerb, which, unlike Herceptin, is not an antibody, but a kinase inhibitor, may be used alone or in combination with Herceptin or chemotherapy. The most common side effects are an acne-like rash and diarrhea.

Herceptin, Kaydcyla, and Perjeta have similar mechanisms of action and hence, similar side effects, including heart damage. Because these drugs can cause heart damage, doctors often check your heart function before treatment, and again while you are taking the drug. Let your doctor know if you develop symptoms such as shortness of breath, leg swelling, and severe fatigue.

Therapies for Estrogen Receptor Positive Cancer

These drugs are used for women who are postmenopausal (or who are premenopausal and have received ovarian suppression therapy) to make hormonal therapies more effective. Drugs include:

- **Ibrance (palbociclib):** This drug inhibits enzymes called cyclin-dependent kinases (CDK4 and CDK6) and is used after an estrogen receptor-positive breast cancer in a postmenopausal woman becomes resistant to hormonal therapy. It may be used along with an aromatase inhibitor such as Femara (letrozole), Aromasin (exemestane), or Arimidex (aromasin), or with the anti-estrogen drug Faslodex (fulvestrant.) The most common side effects are low blood cell counts and fatigue. Nausea and vomiting, mouth sores, hair loss, diarrhea, and headache are less common side effects. Very low white blood cell counts can increase the risk of serious infection.

- **Afinitor (everolimus):** This drug blocks a protein in the body known as mTOR. Affinitor is usually used for an estrogen receptor positive and HER 2 negative tumor after it becomes resistant to an aromatase inhibitor. Common side effects of everolimus include mouth sores, diarrhea, nausea, feeling weak or tired, low blood counts, shortness of breathe, and cough. Everolimus can also increase cholesterol, triglycerides, and blood sugars, so your doctor will check your blood work periodically while you are taking this drug. It can also increase your risk of serious infections, so your doctor will watch you closely for infection.

Targeted therapy for women with BRCA gene mutations

Drugs known as PARP inhbitors are used for women with BRCA1 and BRCA2 gene mutations. They come in pill form and include Lynparza (olaparib) and Talzenna (talazoparib). PARP proteins normally help repair damaged DNA inside cells. The BRCA genes (BRCA1 and BRCA2) also help repair DNA (in a slightly different way), but mutations in one of those genes can stop this from happening. PARP inhibitors work by blocking the PARP proteins. Because tumor cells with a mutated BRCA gene already have trouble repairing damaged DNA, blocking the PARP proteins often leads to the death of these cells.

Olaparib and talazoparib can be used to treat metastatic, HER2-negative breast cancer in women with a BRCA mutation who have already gotten chemotherapy. Olaparib can also be used in women who have already received hormone therapy if the cancer is hormone receptor-positive.

Side effects can include nausea, vomiting, diarrhea, fatigue, loss of appetite, taste changes, low red blood cell counts (anemia), low platelet counts, low white blood cell counts, belly pain, and muscle and joint pain. Rarely, some people treated with a PARP inhibitor have developed a blood cancer, such as myelodysplastic syndrome or acute myeloid leukemia (AML).

Targeted Therapies for Triple Negative Breast Cancer

Tumors that are estrogen receptor negative, progesterone receptor negative, and HER 2 negative result in what's known as triple negative breast cancer. This form can be more of a challenge to treat, as hormonal therapies and HER 2 therapies are usually ineffective.

In some cases, the targeted therapy Avastin (bevacizumab) may be considered. It is classified as an angiogenesis inhibitor. The term angiogenesis means "new blood" and refers to the new blood vessels which need to form to allow cancers to grow. Angiogenesis inhibitors work by preventing cancers from growing new blood vessels, and essentially "starve" the cancer.

One 2018 study found that Avastin, when used in conjunction with chemotherapy, may provide a significant improvement in women with triple negative breast cancer that has spread to the chest wall.

Avastatin, in addition to the side effects common to some of these drugs—such as nausea, diarrhea, and low blood counts—can also cause hemorrhaging and gastrointestinal perforation in rare cases, making its use controversial.

Nutrition & Physical Activity

It's important for you to take very good care of yourself before, during, and after cancer treatment.

- Make healthy living a priority in your daily life.
- Taking care of yourself includes eating well and staying as active as you can.
- Do your best to eat the right amount of calories to maintain a good weight.
- Adequate protein can help to keep up your strength.

What if I don't feel well enough to eat much of anything?

Eating well may actually help you feel better and have more energy. Sometimes, especially during or soon after treatment, you may not feel like eating. Some treatments can leave you feeling tired and uncomfortable. Or you may find that some foods don't taste as good as they used to.

In addition, the side effects of treatment (such as poor appetite, nausea, vomiting, or mouth blisters) can make it hard to eat well. On the other hand, some women treated for breast cancer may have a problem with weight gain.

Your doctor, a registered dietitian, or another healthcare provider can suggest ways to help you meet your nutrition needs and remain as close to a healthy weight as you can.

Is It Okay To Continue To Exercise During Breast Cancer Treatments?

Many women find that they feel better when they stay active. Walking, yoga, swimming, and other activities can keep you strong and increase your energy. Exercise may reduce nausea and pain and make treatment easier to handle. It also can help relieve stress. Whatever physical activity you choose, be sure to talk to your doctor before you start. Also, if your activity causes you pain or other problems, be sure to let your doctor or nurse know this.

Follow-Up Care

What Happens When My Cancer Treatment Rounds Are Complete?

You'll need regular check-ups after treatment for breast cancer. Check-ups help ensure that any changes in your health are noted and treated if needed. If you have any new health problems between checkups, you should contact your doctor.

What Happens At Breast Cancer Follow-Up Appointments?

Your doctor will check for return of the breast cancer. Also, check-ups help detect health problems that can result from cancer treatment.

Check-ups usually include an exam of the neck, underarm, chest, and breast areas. Since a new breast cancer may develop, you should continue to have regular mammograms. You probably won't need a mammogram of a reconstructed breast or if you had a mastectomy without reconstruction. Your doctor may order other imaging procedures or lab tests. You should report any changes in the treated area or in your other breast to your doctor right away.

Breast cancer prevention

Breast cancer prevention starts with healthy habits — such as limiting alcohol and staying active. Understand how to reduce your breast cancer risk.

If you're concerned about developing breast cancer, you might be wondering if there are steps you can take to help prevent breast cancer. Some risk factors, such as family history, can't be changed. However, there are lifestyle changes you can make to lower your risk.

What can I do to reduce my risk of breast cancer?

Research shows that lifestyle changes can decrease the risk of breast cancer, even in women at high risk. To lower your risk:

- **Limit alcohol.** The more alcohol you drink, the greater your risk of developing breast cancer. The general recommendation — based on research on the effect of alcohol on breast cancer risk — is to limit you to less than one drink a day, as even small amounts increase risk.

- **Don't smoke.** Evidence suggests a link between smoking and breast cancer risk, particularly in premenopausal women.

- **Control your weight.** Being overweight or obese increases the risk of breast cancer. This is especially true if obesity occurs later in life, particularly after menopause.

- **Be physically active.** Physical activity can help you maintain a healthy weight, which helps prevent breast cancer. Most healthy adults should aim for at least 150 minutes a week of moderate aerobic activity or 75 minutes of vigorous aerobic activity weekly, plus strength training at least twice a week.

- **Breast-feed**. Breast-feeding might play a role in breast cancer prevention. The longer you breast-feed, the greater the protective effect.

- **Limit dose and duration of hormone therapy**. Combination hormone therapy for more than three to five years increases the risk of breast cancer. If you're taking hormone therapy for menopausal symptoms, ask your doctor about other options. You might be able to manage your symptoms with non-hormonal therapies and medications. If you decide that the benefits of short-term hormone therapy outweigh the risks, use the lowest dose that works for you and continue to have your doctor monitor the length of time you're taking hormones.

- **Avoid exposure to radiation and environmental pollution**. Medical-imaging methods, such as computerized tomography, use high doses of radiation. While more studies are needed, some research suggests a link between breast cancer and cumulative exposure to radiation over your lifetime. Reduce your exposure by having such tests only when absolutely necessary.

Can a healthy diet prevent breast cancer?

Eating a healthy diet might decrease your risk of some types of cancer, as well as diabetes, heart disease and stroke. Consume only Flax oil as oil. Avoid all margarine, vegetable shortenings that contain hydrogenated fats. Reject frozen and preserved meat. Fresh meat is OK. No frozen food and no bakery products. Eat organic diet. Prepare fruit juices yourself. Cheese and potatoes are OK. Maintaining a healthy weight also is a key factor in breast cancer prevention.

Is there a link between birth control pills and breast cancer?

There's some evidence that hormonal contraception, which includes birth control pills and IUDs that release hormones, increases the risk of breast cancer. But the risk is considered very small, and it decreases after you stop using hormonal contraceptives.

A recent study that showed an association between hormonal contraceptive use and breast cancer determined one additional breast cancer could be expected for every 7,690 women who use hormonal contraception for at least one year.

Discuss your contraceptive options with your doctor. Also consider the benefits of hormonal contraception, such as controlling menstrual bleeding, preventing an unwanted pregnancy, and reducing the risk of other cancers, including endometrial cancer and ovarian cancer.

What else can I do?

Be vigilant about breast cancer detection. If you notice any changes in your breasts, such as a new lump or skin changes, consult your doctor. Also, ask your doctor when to begin mammograms and other screenings based on your personal history.

Brassiere – A friend or a foe?

"Dressed to Kill" is a 1995 book by Sydney Ross Singer and Soma Grismaijer that proposes a link between brassiere and breast cancer, which unfortunately is not mentioned in the media for various reasons. It is discussed in the study by the anthropologists Sydney Ross Singer and Soma Grismaijer. Both investigated a total of 4,700 women and they found that the chance of getting breast cancer is 125 times greater for women who wear a brassiere 24 hours a day, than it is for women who do not wear a brassiere. At 12 hours a day the chance is still 21 times greater. The reason for this is not known. Probably the fact that brassieres permanently block lymphatic vessels plays a significant role. Also the changes of the magnetic field through the mostly artificial fibers of the brassier could be responsible for this. Today we still do not know why brassieres have such negative effects, but after this study every woman should reconsider whether she wants to wear a brassiere in the future, or what kind she would like to wear.

Japan has the lowest incidence of breast cancer in the world, and upbringing, nutrition, and many other influences are discussed internationally in an effort to determine why this is so. However the fact is that Japanese women wear fewer brassieres due to smaller breast size, this is at least one reason of perhaps many, but it could also be the main reason for the lower incidence of breast cancer in Japan.

Guide to Breast Self-Examination

Breast self-examination (BSE) is to be performed each month in addition to an annual mammogram or a clinical exam. Knowing your cyclical changes, what is normal for you, and what regular monthly changes in the breast feel like is the best way to keep an eye on your breast health.

This step-by-step, illustrated guide to BSE is easy. It should only take you 15 minutes—once every month. Breast tissue extends from under your nipple and areola up toward your armpit. So you will need a mirror which lets you see both breasts, a pillow for your head and shoulders, and some privacy.

Keep It Regular

If you are pre-menopausal, set a regular time to examine your breasts a few days after your period ends, when hormone levels are relatively stable and breasts are less tender.

If you are already menopausal (have not had a period for a year or more), pick a particular day of the month to do the exam and then repeat your BSE on that day each month.

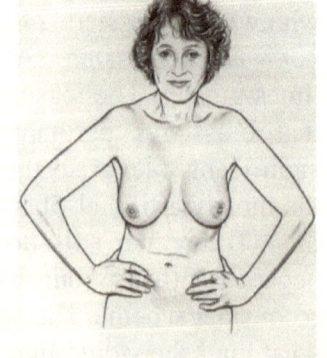

Hands on Hips

Strip to the waist and stand before a mirror. You will need to see both breasts at the same time. Stand with your hands on your hips and check the appearance of your breasts.

Look at the size, shape, and contour. Note changes, if any, in the skin color or texture. Look at the nipples and areolas to see how healthy they look.

Arms Over Your Head

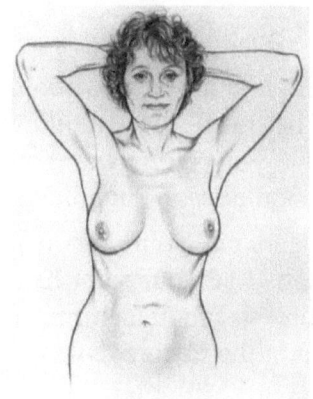

Still standing in front of the mirror, raise your arms over your head and see if your breasts move in the same way and note any differences. Look at the size, shape, and drape, checking for symmetry.

Pay attention to your nipples and areolas to see if you have any dimples, bumps, or retraction (indentation). Look up toward your armpits and note if there is any swelling where your lymph nodes are (lower armpit area).

Stand and Stroke

Raise your left arm overhead and use your right-hand fingers to apply gentle pressure to the left breast. Stroke from the top to the bottom of the breast, moving across from the inside of the breast all the way into your armpit area.

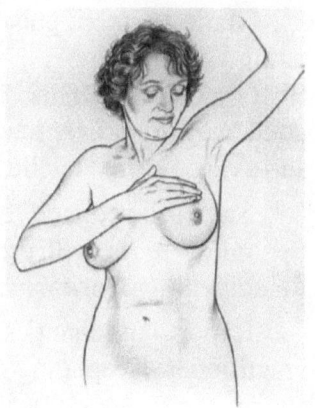

You can also use a circular motion, being sure to cover the entire breast area. Take note of any changes in the texture, color, or size. Switch sides and repeat. This is best done in the shower as wet skin will have the least resistance to the friction of your fingers.

Check Your Nipples

Still facing the mirror, lower both arms. With the index and middle fingers of your right hand, gently squeeze the left nipple and pull forward. Does the nipple spring back into place? Does it pull back into the breast?

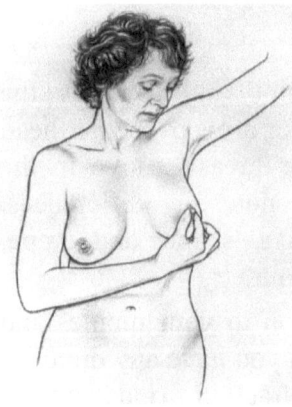

Note whether or not any fluid leaks out. Reverse your hands and check the right nipple in the same way.

Recline and Stroke

This is best done in your bedroom, where you can lie down. Place a pillow on the bed so that you can lie with both your head and shoulders on the pillow.

Lie down and put your left hand behind your head. Use your right hand to stroke the breast and underarm, as you did earlier. Take note of any changes in the texture, color, or size. Switch sides and repeat.

General Tips

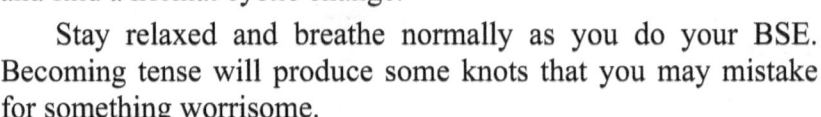

Mark your calendar to remind yourself to do your BSE regularly. This is a good way to prevent worry and find a normal cyclic change.

Stay relaxed and breathe normally as you do your BSE. Becoming tense will produce some knots that you may mistake for something worrisome.

Report any changes or unusual pain to your doctor or nurse practitioner. Keep a log of changes if that helps you remember.

Remember to have an annual clinical exam and a mammogram.

Managing Finances When You Have Breast Cancer

Expenses are probably the last thing you want to think about when you learn you have metastatic cancer. In some ways, it simply doesn't feel fair that people should have to worry about the bottom line financially when facing the physical and emotional turmoil of cancer.

Yet, we live in a world in which cancer is very expensive. In an equation in which expenses go up and ability to work goes down or away entirely, the sum isn't always what we would wish.

While this can sound discouraging, it can make a big difference to take just a few moments to think about your finances early on, and to begin keeping track. It may also help calm some of your fears to learn whether you will need assistance and if so, explore the options that are available.

Tracking Expenses

The most important thing you can do financially is to begin keeping track of your expenses, either when you are diagnosed, or as soon as possible. Many people find it helpful to purchase a notebook devoted only to track your costs. At the same time, you might wish to pick up a folder for holding any important receipts.

This doesn't mean that you need to sit down with an accountant for hours at a time. You have more important things you need to focus on, but a few minutes now could save you and your family time and headaches later on.

Tax Planning

One reason to begin keeping track of costs right away is that many expenses related to cancer are tax deductible. You may be discouraged realizing that medical deductions need to exceed 10 percent of adjusted gross income to qualify, but many people are surprised how quickly this number is reached.

Simply taking the time to record your expenses as they occur (even mileage to your visits is deductible) and dropping receipts in a folder can save countless hours (and money) in the long run.

Budgeting

Once you have your notebook to record your expenses it's helpful to get an idea of your bottom line. This doesn't have to be an intricate spreadsheet detailing all assets and all expenses, but rather a brief sketch of income and debts. This will give you a better idea of whether or not you will have to look into additional options to meet the expenses of your care.

Insurance Concerns

Taking a look at your medical insurance coverage is one of the most important parts of preparing financially when you have metastatic cancer. Here are a few tips:

- **Review your policy** – Most people have a general idea of their medical insurance coverage, but this is a good time to review your policy more closely. This will give you an idea about costs that are covered and whether or not you are underinsured.

- **Understand the difference between in network and out of network providers** – Many insurance policies have different tiers of coverage depending on whether a clinic or hospital is in network or out of network. While a few clinic visits out of network may not add up that much, the cost difference for an out of network hospitalization can add up quickly.

- **Learn about the prior authorization process** – If you find that a treatment you desire is only available out of network, call your insurance company. If you can show that a treatment only available at a higher tier cancer center is superior or has fewer side effects, your insurance may well cover your costs at the in-network rate.

- Keep in mind that these issues need to be figured out before your treatment and this can be frustrating when you're already coping with the symptoms of cancer. If you have a friend or family member who can help you navigate these steps, strongly consider allowing them to help.

- **Review your bills** – It's a good idea to take a moment to review your bills from visits and hospitalizations. Errors are very common and are easier to rectify if discovered early on.

- Review your coverage for home care and hospice care – Even if you're feeling well and hoping you won't need these options, take a look to see what coverage you have for both home health care and hospice care. Most plans cover these needs but the particulars can vary significantly.

Disability Insurance

Loss of income is one of the greatest concerns for those facing metastatic cancer. If you have recently been diagnosed with metastatic cancer, it may feel like it is too early to consider disability, but the best time to consider this is long before you need it. You may have disability insurance through your work or through a private policy, or you may need to consider social security disability.

Since the process of applying for social security disability is lengthy, the best time to apply is as soon as you need it. In order to qualify, you will need a physician to sign a form saying that you are unable to work because of a medical condition that is expected to last at least 12 months (or result in death.) Keep in mind that if you continue to do well and decide you are later able to work, you can always discontinue the program.

You may be confused with the difference between social security disability (SSD) and supplemental security income (SSI). The difference is that SSD is provided for those who have accumulated a specific number of work hours, while SSI is available to those who are low-income or have not worked outside the home enough to earn the work credits needed to qualify.

Financial Support

Even with good insurance coverage, the costs of cancer treatment can be tremendous. By looking at your bottom line as noted, you will have a better idea of whether or not you will need extra support.

Exploring options for financing your treatment

If you don't have the cash you need in the bank—as a large number of people with metastatic cancer do not—take a moment to think about what options you may have. For example:

- Could you take out a loan on your life insurance policy?
- Could you take out a second (or third) mortgage on your home? For those over the age of 65, could you take out a reverse mortgage?
- Do you have any friends or family members who would be willing to loan you money?
- Can you tap into your retirement income? You may need to take a loss, but in the long run, a loss such as this up front may save money down the line.
- Do you have any valuables you would be willing to part with that you could sell?
- Do you have any friends who would be willing to plan a fundraiser in your community or online? Fundraisers are a very common way for people with metastatic breast cancer to raise funds and is usually very effective. There are many online options through social media that you could explore. If you have a friend who enjoys organizing fundraisers, it's amazing how many businesses in most communities will gladly donate services, meals, or other items for a silent auction.

You may think of additional options, but taking a moment to think through some of these possibilities may give you some reassurance.

Financial Assistance

If you're still in the red after evaluating your options, you may wish to check into the various types of assistance available.

There are several organizations which provide assistance for people coping with metastatic breast cancer, though the types of assistance vary. Some offer help with rent or transportation. Others offer financial assistance for childcare. Yet others offer college scholarships for children of those with metastatic breast cancer.

Prescription drug assistance programs may offer you the chance to receive your treatments or medications at discount. There are even free flight programs for cancer patients in some regions.

Since there is such a wide array of options, a great way to get started is by talking to your cancer center social worker. Most cancer social workers have helped others like you find the help they need. You may also wish to enlist an energetic friend or family member to research options for assistance, as this can be a time consuming and tedious task.

Breast Cancer in Young Women

Decision-Making and Coping

Finding Support When You Have Breast Cancer in Your 20s and 30s

Most people have heard that breast cancer can occur in young women, those in their 20s or 30s, or even younger. Yet if you happen to be that young woman, you might feel very alone. Breast cancer isn't supposed to happen when you are at an age when you have young children or are just beginning to think about having children.

Not only does breast cancer come as a shock to many young women, but breast cancer at a young age opens a plethora of issues that aren't faced by women who are older. These issues range from fertility to coping with premature menopause, to coping with the late effects of the disease that may take decades to appear.

On top of this, breast cancer can be a very different disease in young women. We are learning that many of these cancers differ biologically from those found in older women. This translates to differences in everything from treatments to prognosis.

Let's talk about the ways in which living with breast cancer is different for young women than older women, the unique issues younger women face, and how you can find support as a young woman with breast cancer.

Breast Cancer in Young Women

In talking about breast cancer in young women, it's helpful to first define who we are talking about. The definition of "young women" with breast cancer varies by the study or discussion. Many studies talk of women that are aged 40 and under, whereas others talk about women who are under the age of 35. Still others refer to any women who are pre-menopausal at the time of diagnosis, with the average age of menopause being 51.

Amidst all of the pink ribbons, many people believe women with breast cancer get tremendous support. Unfortunately, however, there are many needs that are still unmet for women living with breast cancer, especially those who are young or have metastatic breast cancer.

How Common Is It?

At the current time, roughly a third of women are diagnosed with breast cancer prior to menopause, and 7 percent of breast cancers are diagnosed before the age of 40. Only around 1 percent of breast cancers, however, occur before the age of 30.

Of cancers that occur in women between the age of 15 and 39, breast cancer accounts for around 40 percent of these. In numbers, around 25,000 women under the age of 45 are diagnosed with breast cancer each year, and 2,500 will die.

(Men develop breast cancer too, though breast cancer in men tends to occur later in life, with the average age being around 70.)

Age of breast cancer diagnosis also varies by race. Whereas white women carry a higher risk of breast cancer than black women in the post-menopausal period, breast cancer in black women is twice as common as in whites among those 35 and under, and these women are three times as likely to die from the disease.

Pregnancy-Associated Breast Cancer

One of the heart-breaking aspects of breast cancer in young women is that it is sometimes associated with pregnancy. Breast cancer occurs in around 1 in 3000 pregnancies, and pregnancy-associated breast cancer (cancer during pregnancy and the year or two following pregnancy) accounts for around 7 percent of breast cancers in young women.

The association of breast cancer with pregnancy is confusing, as the effect of pregnancy on the risk of breast cancer is different depending on age. We know that having children earlier in life, and having more children, is associated with a lower risk of developing breast cancer later on. In contrast, having children earlier and having more children is associated with an increased risk of breast cancer in the young, due to the elevation in breast cancer risk following pregnancy. In other words, pregnancy results in an increased risk of breast cancer for the first several years following delivery, but is associated with a lower risk of the disease later on.

How Is Breast Cancer Different in Young Women?

There are many ways in which breast cancer is different in young women than older women. Let's take a look at the differences in symptoms and diagnosis, how breast cancers are biologically different, and how the treatments and prognosis for the disease differ.

Symptoms & Diagnosis of Breast Cancer in Young Women

The most common symptoms of breast cancer in young versus older women come down to a lack of an effective breast cancer screening method for young women. While women who are 40 and over may have screening mammograms, we do not have a widespread effective tool for finding the disease in those under the age of 40. (Women at an increased risk due to family history may begin screening mammograms early or undergo screening breast MRI studies.)

Around four out of five young women with breast cancer are diagnosed after they find a breast lump. In contrast, breast cancer in older women is often found on a mammogram. Even when younger women do have mammograms, these studies are less accurate due to the increased breast density in younger women.

The diagnosis of breast cancer is made in 80 percent of young women after they find a breast lump. For this reason, the diagnosis of breast cancer is often made at a higher stage in younger women. The diagnosis of breast cancer may also be difficult for young women who are pregnant or breastfeeding as breast changes are often considered normal at first.

Genetics & Causes of Breast Cancer in Young Women

Young women with breast cancer are more likely to have a genetic predisposition to the disease. Women under the age of 35 are much more likely to have other family members with breast cancer than older women.

In one study, roughly half of women who were diagnosed before the age of 30 and had a family history of breast cancer had BRCA1, BRCA2, or TP53 mutations versus only 10 percent of women who did not have a family history. People with Cowden syndrome (PTEN mutations) also have an increased risk for early age breast cancer.

We aren't certain what cause breast cancer in young women, but some of the risk factors which have been identified for premenopausal breast cancer include:

- Recent birth control use - The recent use of oral contraceptives raised the risk of breast cancer in young women by a factor of two.
- A history of mantle field radiation for Hodgkin lymphoma
- Early age of menarche (first period.)
- High intake of red meat

In contrast, high vitamin D levels have been associated with a lower risk of premenopausal breast cancer, as have intense physical activity and a high intake of fruits and vegetables.

Types & Characteristics of Breast Cancer in Young Women

There are significant biological differences (molecular characteristics) between breast cancer found in younger versus older women.

Breast cancers in young women are less likely to be estrogen receptor or progesterone receptor positive. On the other hand, these cancers are more likely to be HER2 positive.

Premenopausal breast cancers are also more likely to have a higher tumor grade (for example, are more likely to be grade 3 than grade 1 or 2). Tumor grade is a measure of the aggressiveness of a tumor, so tumors in young women tend to be more aggressive. Triple negative breast cancer, the most difficult breast cancer to treat, is also more common in young women. In one study, 56 percent of black and 42 percent of white women between the ages of 20 and 34 had triple negative tumors.

Treatment

The treatment options for breast cancer in young women can differ from those in older women in some important ways, not only because the molecular characteristics (for example, estrogen positive versus estrogen receptor negative) differ, but also because of menopausal status and the risk of long-term complications.

Surgery

One of the decisions women with early stage breast cancer make is choosing between a lumpectomy and a mastectomy. While decision making in this realm is difficult enough for those who are postmenopausal, it can be terribly confusing for young women. Breast-conserving surgery such as a lumpectomy carries less emotional impact for young women, but at the same time, young women are at a greater risk for recurrence (which is higher with a lumpectomy than a mastectomy). This is a decision that requires careful contemplation for anyone, especially young women.

The decision about having a bilateral mastectomy also becomes more important, as the risk of contralateral breast cancer (developing cancer in the other breast) is fairly common. Women who are treated for early stage breast cancer under the age of 36 have a 13 percent chance of developing cancer in the other breast during the following 10 years.

Chemotherapy

Compared to older women, younger women are more likely to have a recurrence, and adjuvant chemotherapy (chemo after surgery) can decrease this risk. At the same time, however, side effects including premature menopause and more can be more severe for young women, and long term side effects play a larger role.

Hormone Therapy

As noted above, young women are less likely than older women to have estrogen receptor positive tumors reducing the chances that hormone therapy for breast cancer will be effective in young women. For young women who do have estrogen receptor positive tumors, tamoxifen is usually needed instead of an aromatase inhibitor.

We are learning that treatment with an aromatase inhibitor for 5 years (and probably for at least 10) can significantly reduce local recurrences and that this treatment may be more effective than tamoxifen. Unfortunately, aromatase inhibitors can only be used for postmenopausal women. For this reason, younger women often have to consider ovarian suppression therapy. Removal of the ovaries (oophorectomy) or more commonly, treatment with drugs that suppress ovarian function are effective.

Targeted Therapy

On a positive note since HER2 positive tumors are slightly more common in young women, three are now several HER2 targeted therapies (such as Herceptin) available. With the approval of these therapies, the National Cancer Institute upgraded their prognosis for stage I to stage III HER2 positive breast cancer from fair to good.

Radiation Therapy

Radiation therapy can be effective for young women as well. The long-term side effects of radiation therapy, however, become more of an issue.

Long Term Effects

Since young women, in general, are expected to live much longer than older women with the disease, and because some long term effects take many years to develop, these long-term effects may play a larger role for young women with breast cancer:

- Long-term side effects of chemotherapy such as peripheral neuropathy and premature menopause can lead to other medical conditions. The combination of chemotherapy and especially aromatase inhibitors can result in low bone density, osteoporosis, and fractures. A discussion about bone density is particularly important for young women with the disease.

- Long-term side effects of radiation therapy include the risk of secondary cancers—cancers that develop due to the carcinogenic effect of radiation. Women under the age of 50 with breast cancer have a significantly higher risk of secondary cancers including cancers of the bone, ovary, thyroid, kidney, lung, leukemia and lymphoma.

Prognosis

Unfortunately, the survival rate for young women with breast cancer is lower than that for older women with the disease. In a large study of over 200,000 women with breast cancer, women less than 40 are 39 percent more likely to die from their disease. Not only is survival lower, but the improvement in survival rate since 1975 is less than that of older women with the disease.

Part of this disparity is that we do not have a screening test to detect breast cancer early in young women and as noted, the condition is diagnosed in most young women after finding a breast lump. There are other factors as well. When breast cancer recurs in younger women it is more likely to be a metastatic recurrence than a local recurrence.

On a positive note, however, young women do have some advantages. Young women tend to be healthier with fewer other medical conditions. In addition, young women can often better tolerate treatments.

In the past, it was thought that pregnancy-associated breast cancer (breast cancer which develops during pregnancy and in the 5 years following pregnancy) was associated with a poor prognosis. A 2013 study found that women with pregnancy-associated breast cancer had a significantly lower overall survival rate. A 2016 study, in contrast, found that these cancers had a higher risk of local recurrence but did not differ in overall survival rates from non-pregnancy-associated cancers.

Fertility & Contraception

Both wondering if you will be able to get pregnant, and wondering how to prevent getting pregnant are large concerns for young women with breast cancer.

Chemotherapy is well known for throwing a woman smack into menopause, and ovarian suppression therapy may be added as well. For those who want to have kids in the future, there are options for preserving your fertility. Unlike freezing sperm, freezing eggs is still an investigational procedure. That said, freezing embryos is commonly done. Learn more about how breast cancer affects fertility and what your options are for preserving your fertility.

The flip side of this concern is that some people remain fertile even during treatment. For those who have used oral contraceptives, these are no longer an option due to the estrogen in the pills. Other methods of contraception such as condoms or an IUD are instead recommended.

Menopausal Symptoms & Sexual Side Effects

Menopausal symptoms can be extremely annoying for young women being treated for breast cancer. Rather than the typical gradual onset of hot flashes typical of menopause, these symptoms can come on seemingly instantly after chemotherapy begins.

Sexual side effects are common with lower estrogen levels, and these can be particularly bothersome for young women. Talk to your doctor if you are experiencing any of these symptoms. Fortunately, this aspect of life quality is being addressed much more often by oncologists, and there are many options for help.

Coping as a Young Parent

Coping as a young mother (or father) with breast cancer is one of the many differences between support needs in young women versus older women with breast cancer. The lovely self-care brochures which depict women relaxing in a chair and listening to soothing music after chemotherapy may seem entirely fictional if you have toddlers running around using the couch you are sitting on for gymnastics practice.

Being involved in a breast cancer community with other young mothers can be valuable, and may give you many ideas. It's also important to reach out to your family and friends and ask for help. It's easy to forget the busyness of a household with young children when your children are old enough to take care of themselves. Describing a typical day for you may serve as a reminder to older moms you know, motivating them to step in and help as they recall the challenges of young motherhood even without breast cancer.

Emotional Concerns: Anxiety & Depression

Coping with the emotions of breast cancer is difficult for anyone of any age. Yet those who are young have an increased risk of both severe anxiety and depression. At the same time that these emotions occur, having the time to address them may seem overwhelming. Talking with a cancer therapist can be very helpful and has been correlated with improved survival rates for people with breast cancer.

Finding Support

Many people mistakenly believe that there is ample support for women coping with breast cancer, yet this is untrue, especially for those who have "less common" circumstances, such as those who are young. What types of support are available?

Support Groups & Support Communities

Support groups and communities can make a tremendous difference for women (and men) with breast cancer. A caveat, however, is that it's helpful to find a group made up of other young women. The issues you are facing as a young woman are considerably different from those a woman of 60 or 70 may be facing. Women who are grandmothers don't generally share the same concern about the middle of the night feedings during chemotherapy or whether or not it is wise to become pregnant after treatment.

Fortunately, there are many support groups and online communities designed specifically for young women with breast cancer. It can be somewhat challenging finding these groups, but this has been made easier now with hashtags. If you are on Twitter or Facebook and are searching for these groups, use the hashtag #BCSM which stands for breast cancer social media.

Can I Refuse Breast Cancer Treatment?

Making an Informed Choice to Decline Care

One of the central tenets of patient-centered care is informed consent. Informed choice dictates that people have the right to make decisions about the direction of their health care even if that decision is to terminate treatment or seek alternative therapies. This applies as much to everyday ailments like the flu as much as it does serious ones like breast cancer.

Unless you are a minor or are deemed medically incompetent in a court of law—situations that rarely occur with breast cancer—no one but you can determine what is or what is not in your best interest. Even if you decide that the best treatment is no treatment at all.

Reasons to Refuse Treatment

Most people would consider it "normal" to want to seek treatment for breast cancer the moment you are diagnosed, particularly at a time where survival rates are ever-increasing. But this would also infer that not seeking treatment is "abnormal," and that's rarely the case.

There are a plethora of reasons why a woman may not be willing to pursue or continue breast cancer treatment. Some may be transient and simply require a period of adjustment to overcome doubts or fears. Others are fully committed and made with a complete understanding of the implications of the refusal.

Among some of the more common reasons for the refusal of breast cancer treatment:

- **A period of adjustment** - No one really knows how they will respond to a cancer diagnosis until they get one. Some people will panic, others will become resolute, and others still will need time to come terms with the diagnosis before moving forward.

- **Denial** - Even if a woman is in denial, the denial is usually self-protective, allowing her to manage her emotions until she is better able to process the news. Even if she is never able to come to terms with the diagnosis, she is in no way "incompetent." A conscious refusal to act is as much a right as the decision to seek alternative therapy.

- **Personal priorities** - You might assume that cancer would be the number one priority in a person's life, but not everyone agrees. In some cases, a woman may opt to delay treatment for something she considers personally important, such as an upcoming wedding, family trip, or business obligation.

- **Impact on others** - Women are typically nurturers and caregivers in a family. In facing a diagnosis, a woman may worry that the cost of the treatment will bankrupt her family. Or, she may want to spare others from the "horrors" she believes she is going to face, whether real or imagined.

- **Skepticism about health care** - People who have had bad healthcare experiences—or live in economically challenged communities where public service delivery is poor—may have deep-seated skepticism about the medical care offered them.

- **Fear of side effects** - There is no denying that the side effects of cancer therapy can be profound. Sometimes the fear of hair loss, sickness, and pain can become so paralyzing that a woman is unable to see the benefits of treatments for the risks.

- **Matters of faith** - Some religions, like Christian Science, discourage certain medical interventions necessary for cancer treatment. Even if this is not the case, a woman may feel comforted by entrusting her fate to nature or a higher power.

- **Quality of life** - If a woman's prognosis is not good, she may prefer to spend her days doing what she loves rather than fighting a battle she is unlikely to win. Likewise, some women with advanced cancer will choose hospice care with its emphasis on emotional support and pain control rather than aggressive therapeutic interventions that cause pain.

The decision not to be treated is rarely made lightly. According to research from Canada, the majority of women who refused breast cancer therapy were over 50 (53 percent), married (44 percent), and had metastatic disease (61 percent). Of these, 50 percent reported using some form of complementary or alternative medicine.

Role of the Physician

The traditional patriarchal role of the physician has changed vastly in the past 50 or so years. Where doctors were once prescriptive, they are now considered equal partners in your care. When it comes to decisions, however, those are entirely yours.

Within this context, the role of your doctor is to provide you full disclosure of your condition and treatment options in a language you understand. The disclosure would be made without prejudice and coercion. This includes direct coercion (such as calling in a loved one to "talk sense into you") or subtle coercion (telling you "you'll be able to see your grandchildren grow up" if you start treatment).

In theory, the rules of informed consent should always be adhered to without exception. In practice, this is not always the case. Doctors will sometimes try to sway you without even realizing it, often because they believe it is "in your best interest." They might even dismiss complementary or integrative therapies because they either don't believe in them or assert (reasonably) that certain approaches are not evidence-based.

The problem with such dismissals, of course, is that it robs you of the opportunity to fully explore your treatment options. And, in the end, it is far better for your oncologist to know which complementary treatments you are pursuing—and even incorporate them into a treatment plan— to better avoid risks, side effects, and interactions.

What your oncologist is not required to do is engage in unendorsed medical treatments (unless under the auspice of an accredited clinical trial), irrespective of whether the alternative treatment causes direct harm or not.

Beyond that, doctors have no right to implement treatment of any sort without your direct consent.

Exceptions

There are few exceptions to your right to refuse medical treatment. In an emergency situation, doctors do have the right to intervene in order to control the emergency only. Unless there is a legal directive to prevent such treatment, such as a Do-Not-Resuscitate (DNR) order, the doctor has an obligation to intervene, albeit in a specific capacity.

The only other clear exception is parental consent. Parents or legal custodians have the right to approve or deny the medical care of their children up to a certain age (which varies by state). They can also do so for older children who are mentally incapable of making their own decisions even if that child is institutionalized.

That does not mean that doctors cannot legally challenge a parent's decision if they believe it harmful. In fact, medical caretakers have an ethical and legal obligation to advocate for the best interests of a child when parental decisions are potentially dangerous.

The same interventions do not apply to adults. Even a spouse cannot override a partner's refusal of treatment without an extraordinary court action. In such a case, the court would have to declare that woman mentally incompetent and unable to make or carry out important decisions regarding her health.

Even so, the very notion that a court can force a woman with breast cancer to undergo surgery, chemotherapy, or radiation therapy is legally unsound and unheard of in medical practice.

Making an Informed Choice

Most people have encountered one aspect of informed consent, namely the signing of a medical consent form prior to a medical procedure or hospitalization. But informed consent is about more than just signing a document. It involves discussing the potentials risks and benefits of a recommended treatment, as well as the risks and benefits of receiving no treatment.

If, after a reasonable review of the pros and cons, you are not certain whether you want to pursue a treatment, there are several things you should do:

Say so - Tell your doctor that you need time to think about it. Don't just walk away and never come back. Instead, schedule a follow-up appointment where you can discuss any questions that arise. If needed, ask your oncologist for reference materials to better understand the type of breast cancer you have.

Don't feel rushed - Even if you are told your cancer is aggressive, it is not an "emergency" per se. Listen carefully to your prognosis and set aside time to think things through quietly, evaluating what you want and why.

Seek a second opinion - A second opinion is not a rebuke of your oncologist. It is a means to gain assurance or perspective from a neutral party who has looked at your case with fresh eyes. If needed, seek a third or fourth opinion; just be certain you're not looking for someone who will tell you what you want to hear rather than providing you with sound and objective advice.

Separate your anxiety from everyone else's – Often times, the panic we feel is not our own. While you may fully accept your diagnosis, you may find yourself absorbing in the anxiety of others around you. Whatever you decide, the best thing you can do is share your calmness, rather than your frustration, with the ones you love. As much as you'll need their support, they need your support and understanding too.

Reframe the conversation - People will sometimes accuse others of "wanting to die" if they decide to refuse cancer treatment. You can help yourself and others by reframing the conversation, focusing on what you want (such as "I want to enjoy the time we have") rather than what you don't want ("I don't want to feel pain"). By doing so, you're engaging a loved one in conversation rather than a debate.

Keep an open mind - Even if you are at peace with your decision, there may be moments when you have doubts. This is normal. Just because you've come to a decision doesn't mean that it is set in stone. If you find yourself vacillating, consider speaking with a therapist who can help you sort through your emotions

The decision does not need to be made immediately. However, if you do decide to stop or refuse treatment, it is best to inform your doctor rather than dropping off the face of the planet.

Doing so doesn't mean the doctor will suddenly forget you. In many cases, the oncologist will ask you to sign an informed consent document confirming your decision. This not only protects the doctor legally, but it asserts that you fully understand and accept the implications of your choice.

If a Loved One Declines Treatment

If someone you care about has chosen not to continue their cancer treatment, be as supportive as you can. She may have already been met with resistance from her doctors and those closest to her. If her mind is made up, it won't help to add your voice to the debate.

If she is still struggling with her decision, offer to listen and help her sort through the options. Ask if she'd like you to join her at her next doctor's appointment to help her get the answers she needs.

Alternative cancer treatments

We are fighting with cancer since the dawn of history. Every year we discover new diagnostic modalities, better radiotherapy techniques and lots of new chemotherapy drugs. But we have completely failed to defeat this disease called cancer. Think again, are we really going on the right path? Does conventional Medicine really targets upon the prime cause of cancer?

It's not that more effective alternative treatments for cancer don't exist – they most certainly do. It's just that the allopathic system isn't at all interested in divulging real cures. This is because their expensive therapies generate billions of dollars for the cancer industry.

Chemotherapy Doesn't Cure Cancer – It Causes It!

Chemotherapy does, in fact, kill cancer cells. But it also kills healthy cells, along with a patient's immune system and, really, anything else that crosses its path. At worst, such treatments kill patients more quickly than if they had chosen not to undergo them at all.

There's no money to be made in prescribing prevention advice like eating fewer chemicals and exercising more. The "bread and butter" of the cancer industry is unleashing the next, latest-and-greatest cancer drug. Not telling you how to avoid cancer in the first place.

Many people with cancer are interested in trying any treatment that may cure them safely, including complementary and alternative cancer treatments. There is growing evidence that these alternative cancer treatments give wonderful results. Here are some alternative cancer treatments that are very safe and effective.

- **Budwig Protocol -** *The best Alternative Treatment effective in all cancers and all stages with documented 90% success*
- Laetrile (Vitamin B-17) Therapy
- Gerson Therapy
- Dr. Simoncini Baking Soda Cancer Treatment
- High-dose vitamin C
- Frankincense Essential Oil Therapy
- Immunotherapy
- Hyperthermia
- Oxygen Therapy and Hyperbaric Chambers

Laetrile (Vitamin B-17) Therapy

Introduction

During 1950, after many years of research, a dedicated biochemist Dr. Ernest T. Krebs Jr., isolated a new vitamin from bitter apricot kernel that he called 'B-17' or 'Laetrile'. He conducted further lab animal and culture experiments to conclude that laetrile would be effective in the treatment of cancer. As the years rolled by, thousands became convinced that Krebs had finally found the treatment for all cancers. He proposed that cancer was caused by a deficiency of Vitamin B 17 (Laetrile, Amygdaline).

To prove that it was not toxic to humans he injected it into his own arm. As he predicted, there were no harmful or distressing side effects. The Laetrile had no harmful effect on normal cells but was deadly to cancer cells. Dr. Ernst Krebs stated that we need at least a minimum of 100 mg of B-17 or around 7 bitter apricot seeds to almost guarantee a cancer free life.

Nitriloside is a beta-cyanophoric glycosides, a large group of water-soluble, sugar-containing compounds found in a number of plants. Amygdalin is one of the most common nitrilosides. Laetrile is a partly man-made molecule and shares only part of the Amygdalin structure. Both Laetrile and Amygdalin have been promoted as "Vitamin B-17".

Laetrile stands for laevo-rotatory mandelonitrile beta-diglucoside. The "laevo" part references a purified form of B-17 that turns polarized light in a left-turning direction. Dr. Krebs, Jr. believed that only the left-rotating Laevo form was effective against cancer. So it's important to check the purity of your Laetrile.

104

How B-17 works (A tale of two enzymes)

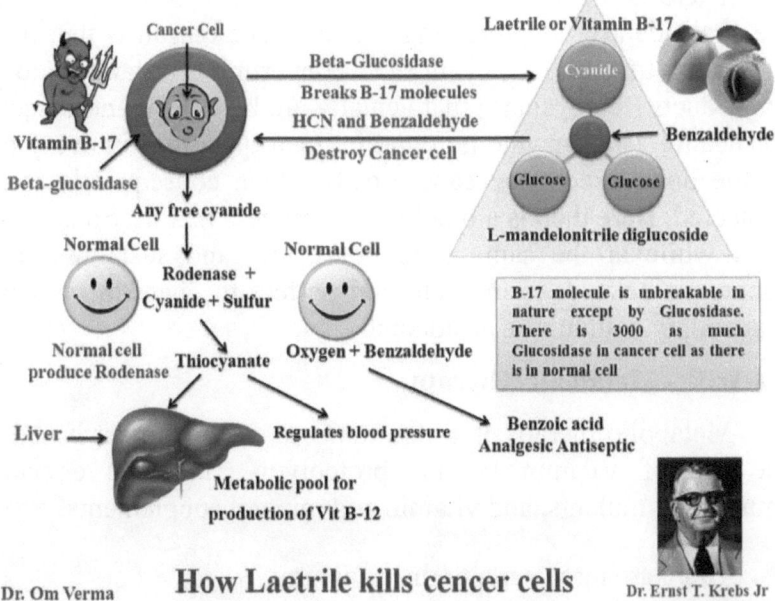

Cancer Cell

Laetrile or Vitamin B-17

Beta-Glucosidase
Breaks B-17 molecules
HCN and Benzaldehyde
Destroy Cancer cell

Cyanide

Benzaldehyde

Vitamin B-17

Beta-glucosidase

Any free cyanide

Normal Cell

Glucose   Glucose

L-mandelonitrile diglucoside

Normal Cell

Rodenase +
Cyanide + Sulfur

Normal cell
produce Rodenase

Thiocyanate

Normal Cell

Oxygen + Benzaldehyde

B-17 molecule is unbreakable in
nature except by Glucosidase.
There is 3000 as much
Glucosidase in cancer cell as there
is in normal cell

Liver →

Regulates blood pressure

Benzoic acid
Analgesic Antiseptic

Metabolic pool for
production of Vit B-12

Dr. Om Verma   **How Laetrile kills cencer cells**   Dr. Ernst T. Krebs Jr

Laetrile, commonly known as Vitamin B-17 or Amygdalin, contains two units of Sugar, one of Benzaldehyde and one of Cyanide, all tightly locked within it. Everyone knows that cyanide can be highly toxic and even fatal if taken in sufficient quantity. However, as it is in locked state is completely inert and absolutely has no effect on living tissue. There is only one substance that can unlock this molecule and release the cyanide. That substance is an enzyme called beta-glucocidase, which we shall call the unlocking enzyme. When B-17 comes in contact with this enzyme, not only the cyanide is released but also Benzaldehyde which is highly toxic by itself. In fact, these two working together are at least 100 times more poisonous to cancer cell than either of them separately. The unlocking enzyme is not found to any dangerous degree anywhere in the body except at the cancer cell where it is present in great quantity. The result is

105

that Vit B-17 is unlocked at the cancer cells becomes poisonous to the cancer cells and only to the cancer cells.

There is another important enzyme called Rodanese, which we shall identify as protecting enzyme. The reason is that it has the ability to neutralize cyanide by converting it instantly into the byproducts (thiocyanate) that actually are beneficial and essential for health. This enzyme is found in great quantities in every part of the body except the cancer cells which consequently is not protected. Here then is a biochemical process that destroys cancer cells while at the same time nourishing and sustaining non-cancerous cells. It is intricate and perfect mechanism of nature that simply couldn't be accidental.

Laetrile - Metabolic Therapy

Metabolic therapy is a non-toxic cancer treatment based on the use of Vitamin B- 17, proteolytic pancreatic enzymes, immuno-stimulants, and vitamin and mineral supplements.

There are three parts to this program:
1. Laetrile
2. Vitamins and enzymes
3. Diet

Phase I Metabolic - Program for the first 21 days

Laetrile

Amygdalin (Laetrile) is available in 500 mg. tablets and in vials (10 cc 3 Gm) for intravenous use. Both forms are used. Two vials of Laetrile are given IV three times weekly for three weeks with at least one day between injections (Mon., Wed., and Fri.). Dose of Amygdalin Tablets 500 mg is 2 tab three times a day with meals on the days on which the patients do not receive the intravenous Laetrile. Thiocyanate levels in the blood can be measured during treatment. In general, the patients who do best are those in whom the thiocyanate level is between 1.2 and 2.5 Mg/DL (Philip E.Binzel).

106

Vitamins and Enzymes

Preven-Ca Caps - Preven-Ca is a comprehensive blend of potent herb and fruit extracts, designed to provide a broad Spectrum of Flavonoids with scientifically demonstrated Antioxidant activity and effectiveness. One capsule with each meal.

Vitamin B15 - One capsule three times a daily at the end of each meal.

Megazyme Forte (Proteolytic Enzymes) Three tablets two hours after each meal (9 daily).

Ester Vitamin C 1000 mg capsule - One capsule with each meal.

Shark Cartilage It has been said that Sharks are the healthiest creature on earth. Sharks are immune to practically every disease known to man. One capsules three times a daily with each meal.

Natural Vitamin E 400 iu - One gel with lunch and one with dinner.

AHCC (Active Hexose Correlated Compound) - Two capsules with each meal.

Multi Vitamin & Mineral Liquid - 1 oz (two tablespoons) once daily with a meal.

Vitamin A & E Emulsion - 5 drops in juice or water three times per day.

Barley Grass Juice - One teaspoon in juice three times per day.

Bitter apricot seeds - No more than 12 every 2 hours 6 times a day.

Dimethyl sulfoxide (DMSO) - DMSO is a by-product of the wood and paper industry. It is known for its ability to permeate living tissue and stimulate cellular processes.

Or Phase 1 Oral

Injectable Amygdalin is replaced with 500mg Amygdalin tablets. Binzel recommends 2 of these tablets with each meal for a total of 6 per day. Otherwise the ORAL Phase 1 includes the same materials as above.

Phase 2 Metabolic - Program for the next 3 months

It comprises the same materials as Phase 1 except that the dosages for the vitamin B-17 as well as the A&E Emulsion Drops change to the following:

Vitamin B-17 500 mg tablets: 1 tablet with each meal and one at bedtime.

Vitamin A & E emulsion drops: 10 drops in juice or water two times per day (suspend for 2 months after 3 months of use).

Diet

Consume those fruits (i.e. seeds), grains and nuts that are rich in laetrile. Consume salads with healthy dressings. For protein patient should consume whole grains including corn, beans, buckwheat, nuts, and dried fruits. Real butter in small amounts is permitted. The patients are not permitted anything which contains white flour or white sugar. Take away all meat, all poultry, all fish, all eggs and milk from patients. Margarine is detrimental to good nutrition. No coffee is permitted.

Zinc acts as transport vehicle for laetrile in the body. If patient does not have sufficient zinc, laetrile will not get into the tissues of the body. That's why you should give a spoonful of pumpkin seeds along with bitter apricot kernels. The body will not rebuild any tissue without sufficient quantities of Vitamin C etc.

The Gerson Therapy

The Gerson Therapy is a natural treatment that activates the body's extraordinary ability to heal itself through an organic, plant-based diet, raw juices, coffee enemas and natural supplements.

With its whole-body approach to healing, the Gerson Therapy naturally reactivates your body's magnificent ability to heal itself – with no damaging side effects. This a powerful, natural treatment boosts the body's own immune system to heal cancer, arthritis, heart disease, allergies, and many other degenerative diseases. Dr. Max Gerson developed the Gerson Therapy in the 1930s, initially as a treatment for his own debilitating migraines, and eventually as a treatment for degenerative diseases such as skin tuberculosis, diabetes and, most famously, cancer.

An abundance of nutrients from copious amounts of fresh, organic juices are consumed every day, providing your body with a super-dose of enzymes, minerals and nutrients. These substances then break down diseased tissue in the body, while coffee enemas aid in eliminating toxins from the liver.

Throughout our lives our bodies are being filled with a variety of carcinogens and toxic pollutants. These toxins reach us through the air we breathe, the food we eat, the medicines we take and the water we drink. The Gerson Therapy's intensive detoxification regimen eliminates these toxins from the body, so that true healing can begin.

How the Gerson Therapy Works

The Gerson Therapy regenerates the body to health, supporting each important metabolic requirement by flooding the body with nutrients from about 15- 20 pounds of organically-grown fruits and vegetables daily. Most is used to make fresh raw juice, up to one glass every hour, up to 13 times per day. Raw and cooked solid foods are generously consumed. Oxygenation is usually more than doubled, as oxygen deficiency in the blood contributes to many degenerative diseases. The metabolism is also stimulated through the addition of thyroid, potassium and other supplements, and by avoiding heavy animal fats, excess protein, sodium and other toxins.

Degenerative diseases render the body increasingly unable to excrete waste materials adequately, commonly resulting in liver and kidney failure. The Gerson Therapy uses intensive detoxification to eliminate wastes, regenerate the liver, reactivate the immune system and restore the body's essential defenses – enzyme, mineral and hormone systems. With generous, high-quality nutrition, increased oxygen availability, detoxification, and improved metabolism, the cells – and the body – can regenerate, become healthy and prevent future illness.

Juicing

Fresh-pressed juice from raw foods provides the easiest and most effective way of providing high-quality nutrition. By juicing, patients can take in the nutrients and enzymes from nearly 15 pounds of produce every day, in a manner that is easy to digest and absorb.

Every day, a typical patient on the Gerson Therapy for cancer consumes up to thirteen glasses of fresh, raw carrot-apple and green leaf juices. These juices are prepared hourly from fresh, raw, organic fruits and vegetables, using a two-step juicer or a masticating juicer used with a separate hydraulic press.

The Gerson Therapy Diet

The Gerson Therapy diet is plant-based and entirely organic. The diet is naturally high in vitamins, minerals, enzymes, micro-nutrients, and extremely low in sodium, fats, and proteins. The following is a typical daily diet for a Gerson patient on the full therapy regimen:

110

- Thirteen glasses of fresh, raw carrot-apple and green-leaf juices prepared hourly from fresh, organic fruits and vegetables.
- Three full plant-based meals, freshly prepared from organically grown fruits, vegetables and whole grains. A typical meal will include salad, cooked vegetables, baked potatoes, Hippocrates soup and juice.
- Fresh fruit and vegetables available at all hours for snacking, in addition to the regular diet.

Supplements

All medications used in connection with the Gerson Therapy are classed as biologicals, materials of organic origin that are supplied in therapeutic amounts. The supplements used on the Gerson Therapy include:
- Potassium compound
- Lugol's solution
- Vitamin B-12
- Thyroid hormone
- Pancreatic Enzymes

Detoxification

Coffee enemas are the primary method of detoxification of the tissues and blood on the Gerson Therapy. Coffee enemas accomplish this essential task, assisting the liver in eliminating toxic residues from the body for good. Cancer patients on the Gerson Therapy may take up to 5 coffee enemas per day. The Gerson Therapy also utilizes castor oil to stimulate bile flow and enhance the liver's ability to filter blood.

Simoncini's Baking Soda Cancer Treatment

Dr. Tullio Simoncini is a medical doctor in Italy who has done more than anyone to explore the uses of the baking soda cancer treatment as an alternative cancer treatment. It is known that cancer creates and favors an acid environment and because of this, Dr. Simoncini and others have used sodium bicarbonate as an alkaline therapeutic agent.

The way that acidity seems to protect cancer is not fully understood. It seems that cytotoxic T-cells, which may attack cancer cells under normal conditions, are inactivated in an acid extracellular fluid. Also, the type of acidity that cancer produces, i.e., lactic acid, stimulates vascular endothelial growth factor and angiogenesis. This is like a highway project, which enables a tumor to build the blood vessels that it needs to bring the nutrients for it to survive. So the tumor creates an environment in which it can then exist comfortably.

Baking Soda's Alkalinity Fights Cancer's Acidity

At a pH of about 10, sodium bicarbonate is an antidote to this acidity. It can be used clinically in sterile, intravenous form. This is a liquid, sterile bicarbonate of soda. The baking soda cancer treatment is well-tolerated, even with frequent repeated dosing. Dr. Simonchini also injects soda bicarb solution directly into the tumors at his center.

Cancer a Fungus problem?

Dr. Simonchini says that cancer is caused by fungus However, it is useful to know that not only does sodium bicarbonate disrupt the comfortable environment of tumors, but it also has anti-fungal effect.

Best Alternative Treatment - Budwig Protocol

90% documented success in all types of Cancers

Bonding of Alpha-Linolenic Acid and Sulfurated Protein

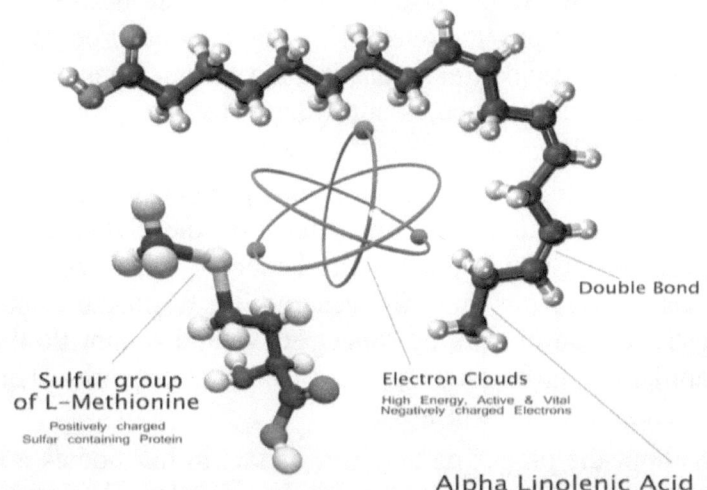

Double Bond

Sulfur group
of L–Methionine
Positively charged
Sulfar containing Protein

Electron Clouds
High Energy, Active & Vital
Negatively charged Electrons

Alpha Linolenic Acid

Dr. Budwig has been referred to as a top European cancer research scientist, biochemist, pharmacologist, and physicist. Dr. Budwig was a seven-time Nobel Prize nominee.

In Germany in 1952, she was the central government's senior expert for fats and pharmaceutical drugs. She's considered one of the world's leading authorities on fats and oils. Her research has shown the tremendous effects that commercially processed fats and oils (having Trans fatty acids) have in destroying cell membranes and lowering the voltage in the cells of our bodies, which then result in chronic and terminal disease including cancer.

What we have forgotten is that we are body electric. The cells of our body fire electrically. They have a nucleus in the center of the cell which is positively charged, and the cell membrane, which is the outer lining of the cell, is negatively charged. We are all aware of how fats clog up our veins and arteries and are the leading cause of heart attacks, but we never

113

looked beyond the end of our noses to see how these very dangerous fats and oils are affecting the overall health of our minds and bodies at the cellular level.

Dr. Budwig discovered that when unsaturated fats have been chemically treated, their unsaturated qualities are destroyed and the field of electrons removed. This commercial processing of fats destroys the field of electrons that the cell membranes (60-75 trillion cells) in our bodies must have to fire properly (i.e. function properly).

The fats' ability to associate with protein and thereby to achieve water solubility in the fluids of the living body is destroyed. As Budwig put it, "the battery is dead because the electrons in these fats and oils recharge it." When the electrons are destroyed the fats are no longer active and cannot flow into the capillaries and through the fine capillary networks. This is when circulation problems arise.

Without the proper metabolism of fats in our bodies, every vital function and every organ is affected. This includes the generation of new life and new cells. Our bodies produce over 500 million new cells daily. Dr. Budwig points out that in growing new cells, there is a polarity between the electrically positive nucleus and the electrically negative cell membrane with its high unsaturated fatty acids. During cell division, the cell, and new daughter cell must contain enough electron-rich fatty acids in the cell's surface area to divide off completely from the old cell. When this process is interrupted the body begins to die. In essence, these commercially processed fats and oils are shutting down the electrical field of the cells allowing chronic and terminal diseases to take hold of our bodies.

A very good example would be tumors. Dr. Budwig noted that "The formation of tumors usually happens as follows. In those body areas which normally host many growth processes, such as in the skin and membranes, the glandular organs, for example, the liver and pancreas or the glands in the stomach and intestinal tract—it is here that the growth processes are brought to

114

a standstill. Because the polarity is missing, due to the lack of electron rich highly unsaturated fat, the course of growth is disturbed—the surface-active fats are not present; the substance becomes inactive before the maturing and shedding process of the cells ever takes place, which results in the formation of tumors."

She pointed out that this can be reversed by providing the simple foods, cottage cheese, and flax seed oil, which revises the stagnated growth processes. This naturally causes the tumor or tumors present to dissolve and the whole range of symptoms which indicate a "dead battery are cured." Dr. Budwig did not believe in the use of growth-inhibiting treatments such as chemotherapy or radiation. She was quoted as saying "I flat declare that the usual hospital treatments today, in a case of tumorous growth, most certainly leads to worsening of the disease or a speedier death, and in healthy people, quickly causes cancer."

Dr. Budwig discovered that when she combined flaxseed oil, with its powerful healing nature of essential electron rich unsaturated fats, and cottage cheese, which is rich in sulfur protein, the bonding produced makes the oil water soluble and easily absorbed into the cell membrane.

I found testimonials of people from around the world who had been diagnosed with terminal cancer (all types of cancer), sent home to die and were now living healthy, normal lives. Not only had Dr. Budwig been using her protocol for treating cancer in Europe, but she also treated other chronic diseases such as arthritis, heart infarction, irregular heartbeat, psoriasis, eczema (other skin diseases), immune deficiency syndromes (Multiple Sclerosis and other autoimmune diseases), diabetes, lungs (respiratory conditions), stomach ulcers, liver, prostate, strokes, brain tumors, brain (strengthens activity), arteriosclerosis and other chronic diseases. Dr. Budwig's protocol proved successful where orthodox traditional medicine was failing.

Prime Cause of Cancer

We are fighting with cancer since the dawn of history. Every year we discover new diagnostic modalities, better radiotherapy techniques and lots of new chemotherapy drugs. But we have completely failed to defeat this disease called cancer. Think again, are we really going on the right path? Does conventional Medicine really targets upon the prime cause of cancer???

Otto Warburg – Biography

Otto Heinrich Warburg (October 8, 1883 – August 1, 1970), son of physicist Emil Warburg, was a German physiologist, medical doctor and Nobel laureate. His mother was the daughter of a Protestant family of bankers and civil servants from Baden. Warburg studied chemistry under the great Emil Fischer, and earned his "Doctor of Chemistry" in Berlin in 1906. He then earned the degree of "Doctor of Medicine" in Heidelberg in 1911. Between 1908 and 1914, Warburg was affiliated with the Naples Marine Biological Station, in Naples, Italy, where he conducted research.

He served as an officer in the elite Uhlan (cavalry regiment) during the First World War, and was given the Iron Cross (1st Class) award for his bravery. Warburg is considered one of the 20th century's leading biochemists. Towards the end of the war, Albert Einstein, who had been a friend of Warburg's father Emil, wrote Warburg asking him to leave the army and return to academia, since it would be a tragedy for the world to lose his talents. Einstein and Warburg later became friends, and Einstein's work in physics had great influence on Otto's biochemical research.

While working at the Marine Biological Station, Warburg performed research on oxygen consumption in sea urchin eggs after fertilization, and proved that upon fertilization, the rate of respiration increases by as much as six fold. His experiments also

116

proved that iron is essential for the development of the larval stage.

In 1918, Warburg was appointed professor at the Kaiser Wilhelm Institute for Biology in Berlin-Dahlem. By 1931 he was promoted as director of the Kaiser Wilhelm Institute for Cell Physiology, which was later on, renamed the Max Planck Society. Warburg investigated the metabolism of tumors and the respiration of cells, particularly cancer cells, and in 1931 was awarded the Nobel Prize in Physiology for his "discovery of the nature and mode of action of the respiratory enzyme."

Nomination for a second Nobel Prize

In 1944, Warburg was nominated for a second Nobel Prize in Physiology by Albert Szent-Györgyi, for his work on nicotinamide, the mechanism and enzymes involved in fermentation, and the discovery of flavin (in yellow enzymes), but was prevented from receiving it by Adolf Hitler's regime.

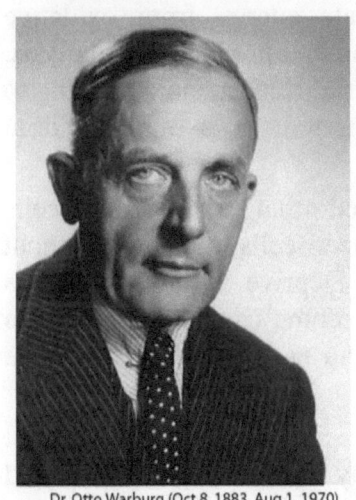

Dr. Otto Warburg (Oct 8, 1883 Aug 1, 1970)

Otto Warburg edited and had much of his original work published in The Metabolism of Tumors and wrote New Methods of Cell Physiology (1962). Otto Warburg was thrilled when Oxford University awarded him an honorary doctorate.

In his later years, Warburg was convinced that illness is resulted from pollution; this caused him to become a bit of a health advocate. He insisted on eating bread made from wheat grown organically on his farm. When he visited restaurants, he often made arrangements to pay the full price for a cup of tea, but to only be served boiling water, from which he would make tea with a tea bag he had brought with him. He was also known to go to significant lengths to obtain organic butter, the quality of which he trusted.

The Otto Warburg Medal

The Otto Warburg Medal is intended to commemorate Warburg's outstanding achievements. It has been awarded by the German Society for Biochemistry and Molecular Biology since 1963. The prize honors and encourages pioneering achievements in fundamental biochemical and molecular biological research. The Otto Warburg Medal is regarded as the highest award for biochemists and molecular biologists in Germany.

Prime cause of Cancer

Warburg hypothesized that cancer growth is caused by tumor cells mainly generating energy (as e.g. adenosine triphosphate / ATP) by anaerobic breakdown of glucose (known as fermentation, or anaerobic respiration). This is in contrast to healthy cells, which mainly generate energy from oxidative breakdown of pyruvate. Pyruvate is an end product of glycolysis, and is oxidized within the mitochondria. Hence, and according to Warburg, cancer should be interpreted as a mitochondrial dysfunction.

In short, Warburg summarized that all normal cells absolutely require oxygen, but cancer cells can live without oxygen - a rule without exception. Deprive a cell 35% of its oxygen for 48 hours and it would become cancerous. **Dr. Otto Warburg clearly mentioned that the root cause of cancer is lack of oxygen in the cells.**

He also discovered that cancer cells are anaerobic (do not breathe oxygen), get the energy by fermenting glucose and produce levo-rotating lactic acid, and the body becomes acidic. Cancer cannot survive in the presence of high levels of oxygen, as found in an alkaline state.

He postulated that sulfur containing protein and some unknown fat is required to attract oxygen into the cell. This fat plays a major role in the respiration and functioning of Warburg respiratory enzyme. He thought it would be butyric acid and made experiment, but this attempt was a failure. For many decades scientists were trying to identify this unknown and mysterious fat but nobody succeeded (Otto Warburg, Wikipedia).

Dr. Johanna Budwig - Biography & Science

Birth of an angel

A lovely couple, Hermann Budwig and Elisabeth, lived in Essen town of Germany situated on the bank of river Ruhr. On the eve of 30th September, 1908 Elisabeth delivered a brilliant and lucky angel. Hermann and 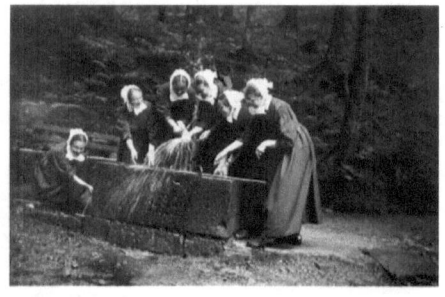 Elisabeth were very happy, and celebrating. They called her Johanna. In German, Johanna means a gift from God. In the family and neighborhood everybody was talking that Johanna is very lucky, she will study in a college and become a big doctor. Actually, 1908 was very fortunate and important year for the freedom of women in Germany. Government for the first time in history, changed laws, and allowed women to study in college and Universities. Also the German parliament passed a legislation to allow women to become members of political parties and prestigious clubs. Though women were given new rights and freedom, liberalization was slow and old values still persisted.

The tough life of a sage of science

Unluckily, Elisabeth died in 1920; family members thought that her father, being a poor loco mechanic, might not look after Johanna. So she was sent to an orphanage. This was a great shock for the little Johanna, but it had one positive side also. Education up to higher level was totally free for orphans.

In 1926, Germany was slowly recovering from the after effects of the First World War. Economic conditions were improving. Scholars and scientists were developing new technologies in every field. One third of all Nobel Prizes were being given to German academics.

Deaconess at Kaiserswerth

Johanna was very intelligent and sharp in studies from the beginning. In order to achieve good future, she decided to join the renowned Deaconess's Institute of Kaiserswerth in 1925. Theodor Fliedner, a pastor, founded Kaiserswerth Institute for welfare of unmarried mothers, prisoners, patients, orphans and poor children in 1836. In the beginning a Hospital and a Nursing School was established. This school was very famous Nursing School of that time.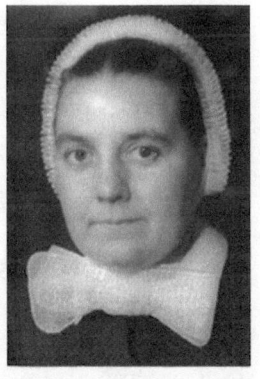
Florence Nightingale, known as mother of modern nursing, also studied in this Deaconess School in 1850. Intelligent Johanna easily got admission in this Institute. She was made a "deaconess" on March 30, 1932. This was the most appropriate place for her. There was a 1000 bedded hospital, pharmacy and a boarding school. She decided to study pharmacy.

After completing preliminary education in Kaiserswerth, she joined Münster University for further studies. Her analytical thinking and precise knowledge was noticed by her Professor Dr Hans Paul Kaufmann. He always encouraged and helped her. Here she passed state examination in pharmacy and was rewarded distinction in chemistry in 1936. Then she continued further education in physics, and received the title "Doctor of Science" at the University of Münster in 1938. On August 1, 1939, she was appointed as in-charge of pharmacy at the Military Hospital in Kaiserswerth.

Next month, Hitler's military forces attacked Poland. During war time, brave Johanna was busy in organizing and expanding the pharmacy. The war was not an easy time. There were two thousand people living in Kaiserswerth. Johanna was responsible for ensuring that there were enough medicines in this time of rationing and a thriving black market. She was well prepared and ready to fulfill any emergency demand for her patients. Many of her fellow deaconesses were often jealous and not co-operating but she continued evolving her professional skills. She was strong and was confronting every opponent (Dr. Johanna Budwig Stiftung).

Dr Budwig's scientific thinking, work and career

After Second World War, Johanna left Kaiserswerth in 1949. Soon Prof. Kaufmann came to know that she had left Kaiserswerth. He immediately met and persuaded her to work with him in Münster University, as he was always impressed from her talent. He converted the basement of his house into a laboratory and arranged all facilities for her research. He was famous as Fat Pope in the whole Europe.

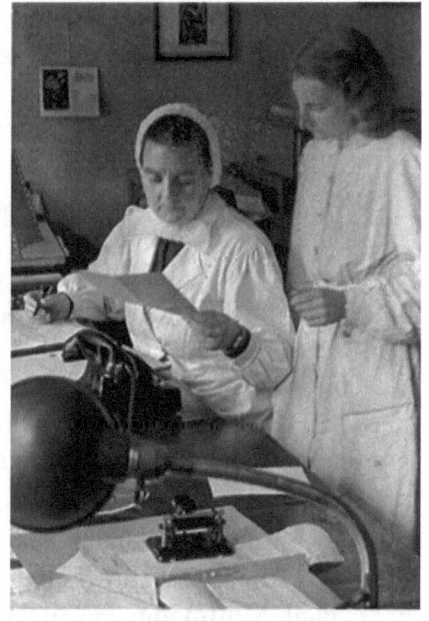

On Prof. Kaufmann's recommendation, Johanna was appointed as the chief expert for drugs and fats at the Federal Institute for Fats Research, Germany. This was the country's largest office issuing the approval of new drugs used for cancer. Many applications had been submitted to her for approval. These were the medications for cancer therapy with the sulfhydryl group (sulfur-containing protein compounds). Everywhere she saw that fats played a role in cellular respiration, also in expert reports provided by well-known professors like Prof. Nonnenbruch. Unfortunately, fats could only be detected in the late stage, and there were no method to distinguish between fats chemically.

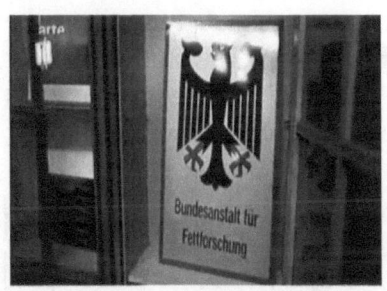

By this time, she developed paper chromatography. With this technique for first time she was able to detect fatty acids and lipoproteins directly even in 0.1 ml of blood. She used Co60 isotopes successfully to produce the first differential reaction for fatty acids, and produced the first direct iodine value via radioiodine. She also developed control of atmosphere in a closed system by using gas systems which act as antioxidants. She further developed Coloring methods, separating effects of fats and fatty acids. She too studied their behavior in blue and red light with fluorescent dyes.

Using rhodamine red dye, she studied the electrical behavior of the unsaturated fatty acids with their "halo". With this technique she could prove that electron rich highly unsaturated Linoleic and Linolenic fatty acids (Flax oil being the richest source) were the mysterious and undiscovered decisive fats required to attract oxygen into the cells, which Otto Warburg could not find. She studied the electromagnetic function of pi-electrons of the linolenic acid in the cell membranes, for nerve function, secretions, mitosis, as well as cell division. She also examined the synergism of the sulfur containing protein with the

pi-electrons of the highly unsaturated fatty acids and their significance for the formation of the hydrogen bridge between fat and protein, which represent "the only path" for fast and focused Transport of electrons during respiration. This research was extensively

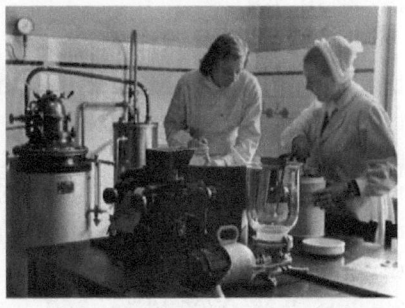

published in 1950 in Neue Wege in der Fettforschung (New Directions in Fat Research) and other publications.

This immediately caused an excitement and turmoil in the scientific community. Everybody thought that it would open new doors in Cancer research. She also proved that hydrogenated fats and refined oils including all Trans-fatty acids were not having vital electrons and were respiratory poisons.

During her research, she found that the blood of seriously ill cancer patients had deficiency of unsaturated essential fats (Linoleic and Linolenic fatty acids), lipoproteins, phosphatides, and hemoglobin. She also had noticed that cancer 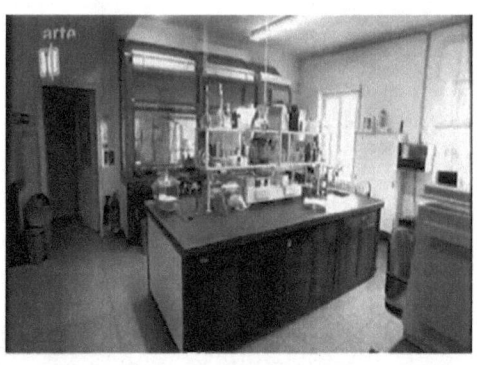 patients had a strange greenish-yellow substance in their blood which is not present in the blood of healthy people (Budwig, Cancer The Problem And The Solution).

She wanted to develop a healing program for cancer. So she enrolled over 642 cancer patients from four hospitals in Münster. She gave Flax oil and Cottage Cheeseto these patients. After just three months, patients began to improve in health and strength, the yellow green substance in their blood began to disappear, tumors gradually receded and at the same time the nutrients began to rise.

This way she developed a simple cure for cancer, based on the consumption of Flax oil with low fat Quark or cottage cheese, raw organic diet, mild exercise, Flax oil massage and the healing powers of the sun. It was a great victory and the first milestone in the battle against cancer. She treated approx. 2500 cancer patients during last few decades. Prof. Halme of surgery clinic in Helsinki used to keep records of her patients. According to him her success was over 90%, and this was achieved in cases, which were rejected by Allopathic doctors.

Dr. Budwig was a courageous scientist. She **loudly and convincingly argued that consumption of highly processed foods, particularly edible oils and margarines, which block the oxidation processes in the cells, are responsible for the development of cancer and other degenerative diseases.** She met with great resistance from food industry giants, who were doing everything to prevent the spread of her sensational discovery. In 1952, under the influence of strong pressure from this lobby, she lost her job and was barred from the research work.

Joins Medical School at Göttingen

Opponents of Dr. Johanna blamed her that she should not treat cancer patients because she doesn't have a doctor's degree. She felt this and eventually joined medical school in Göttingen in

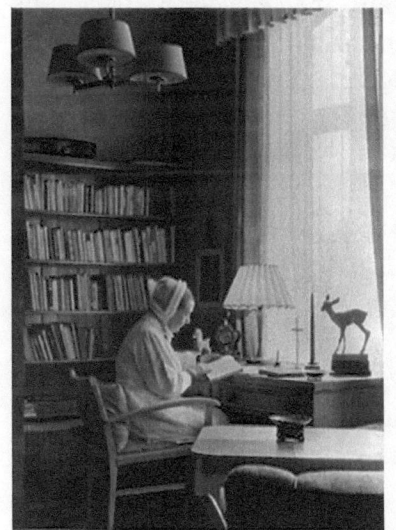

1955. Budwig was 47 years old at that time. She also continued her research work along with her studies. *Budwig successfully treated Prof. Martius's wife, who suffered from Breast Cancer*

One night a woman came with her small child whose arm was supposed to be amputated due to a tumor. She treated her and soon the amputation surgery was dismissed, and the child quickly did very well.

A Swiss woman came to her clinic in Göttingen. She suffered from Colon Cancer with metastasis and intestinal obstruction. Several doctors examined her, and were to be operated on Christmas Eve. On Budwig's request, she was treated by her protocol. The tumor of the colon quickly subsided. Seven weeks later, she was discharged without any detectable tumor. It is interesting that the Swiss custom

125

officer was not ready to believe that the submitted passport belonged to same lady. Her look was so much changed! At home her daughter welcomed saying: "You look healthy, younger and more beautiful (from her book The Death of the Tumor – Vol. II).

After this, University allowed her to treat cancer patients with her oil-protein diet. She was getting miraculous results. University professors were excited with the results, but wanted that she should also include chemo and radiotherapy. She was rigid and didn't want to compromise. So she had differences and conflicts with her professors and ultimately left Göttingen (Budwig, Cancer The Problem And The Solution).

Last Destination - Dietersweiler-Freudenstadt

Eventually, she shifted to Dietersweiler-Freudenstadt, where she lived till her death. There she completed Ph.D. in Naturopathy so that she could legally treat cancer patients. She continued treating her patients in Freudenstadt. In 1968 she created unique Eldi oils for massage and enema, called Electron Differential Oils after performing precise spectroscopic measurements of the light absorption in different oils. *US pain institute has written somewhere: "What this crazy woman does with her ELDI oils, none of us manages to do via pain killers."*

Budwig conducted more than 200 lectures worldwide. Dr. Budwig was popular in the U.S. as FLAX SEED lady from Freudenstadt. She delivered her last public Lecture in Freudenstadt on March 3, 1999. On November 28, 2002, she fell down in her bathroom and got a fracture in right femur neck. She was admitted in a nursing home and ultimately died on May 19, 2003.

Budwig Protocol

The Budwig Protocol is one of the most widely followed alternative treatments for cancer and other diseases. The diet seems simple, but foods are powerful and can heal a person.

Transition Diet

The Transition diet is especially recommended for patients of liver, pancreatic or gall bladder cancers. The basic principle is that for 3 days nothing is eaten and drunk except the following written and at least three times daily warm tea (herbal teas from peppermint, rose hip, mallow or green tea) is drunk. Dr Budwig has recommended variant 1 for patients with a relatively good energy state, and variant 2 and 3 mainly for seriously ill patients.

Variant 1

Variant 1 for three days, 250 g of linomel or alternatively freshly crushed Flax seed is eaten together with the following:

- Freshly pressed fruit juices without added sugar.
- Freshly pressed vegetable juices such as carrot, celery juice, red beetroots and apple juice.
- Chinese tea and black tea are allowed in the morning
- Honey for sweetening is allowed. Just as grape juice for drinking and as a sweetener. Energetically weak patients can also consume sparkling wine and linomel.

Variant 2

For three days, oat meal cereal very hour with linomel is eaten daily with the following juices:

- Freshly pressed fruit juices or freshly pressed vegetable juices such as carrot, celery juice, beetroot and apple juice.
- Chinese tea and black tea are allowed in the morning.
- Honey for sweetening is allowed. Just as grape juice for drinking and as a sweetener.

- Energetically weak patients can also consume sparkling wine and linomel.

Variant 3

For three days, oatmeal soup with linomel is given three times a day together with the following juices:

- Freshly pressed fruit juices or fruit juices without added sugar.
- Freshly pressed vegetable juices such as carrot, celery juice, beetroot and apple juice.
- Chinese tea and black tea are allowed in the morning.
- Honey for sweetening is allowed. Just as grape juice for drinking and as a sweetener.
- Energetically weak patients can also consume sparkling wine and linomel.

It is often experienced frequently that patients mixed all three variants and "nevertheless" had good results. So better you to stick to one variant. (Budwig – Cancer The Problem And The Solution 2005: p.36).

Budwig Diet

The Budwig Protocol is necessary for many diseases from cancer to type 2 diabetes and heart disease to autoimmune diseases, etc. Its purpose is to energize the cells by restoring the natural electrical potential in the cell. Many human diseases are caused by "sick cells" which have lost their normal electrical potential; generally via a lower ATP energy in the cell's mitochondria.

6:00 AM – Sauerkraut juice

A glass of sauerkraut juice consumed before breakfast every morning. It is rich in vitamins including C, enzymes and helps develop the health-promoting gut flora. Sauerkraut is cabbage that has been pickled by natural fermentation, mainly with lactobacillus bacteria. It is slightly salty, sharp and sour. Well made, it is much nicer than it sounds. You may also consume another glass of sauerkraut juice later in the day.

It interesting that sauerkraut contains right rotating lactic acids and is highly alkaline and neutralizes levo-rotating lactic acids and makes our body alkaline. That is why Marcus Porcius Cato the Elder issued a statement - Carcinomas are incurable except with the treatment with Sauerkraut.

8:00 AM Breakfast

Green or herbal tea

Start breakfast with a cup of warm herbal or green tea. Sweeten with only natural honey. You can add lemon or grape juice. Patient should take such a tea before or with Linomel Muesli. You may consume 4-5 such teas in a day.

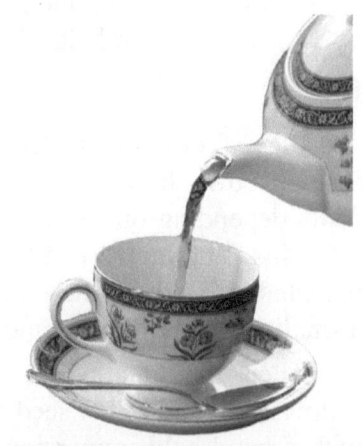

Linomel Muesli or Oil-Protein Muesli

This should be made fresh and consumed within 15 minutes. It is full of high energy pi-electrons, attract oxygen in the cells

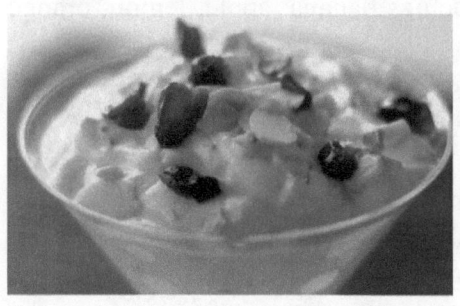

and capable of healing cell membranes. It is full of energy-rich omega-3 fats, has power to attract healing photons from sun through resonance. As "Om" is divine word and synonym of God in India. According to Hindu Mythology, the whole universe is located inside "Om", so the name Omkhand has been given to this wonderful recipe in Hindi.

Ingredients

- 3 Tbsp cold pressed organic Flax seed oil (FO)
- 100-125gm (6 Tbsp) Quark or Cottage Cheese(CC)

- 2 Tbsp freshly ground Flax seeds
- 2 Tbsp milk
- 1 cup fruits
- ¼ cup dried nuts
- Natural honey
- Flavorings – lemon, apple cider vinegar, cinnamon, pure cacao, natural vanilla, shredded coconut etc.

Recipe

Place 2 tablespoons Linomel or freshly ground Flax seeds in a small bowl. It is covered with raw, crushed or diced seasonal fruits depending on the season. Pour some orange or grape juice over this. Linomel^{Tm} is a brand name and originally created and patented by Budwig. It is a cereal made from cracked Flax Seed, a small amount of honey and a little milk powder.

Then the Quark-Flax seed oil cream is prepared in as follows: First add Flax seed oil, milk and honey and blend briefly with a hand-held immersion electric blender, then gradually add the Quark in smaller portions. Blend till oil and Quark is thoroughly mixed with no separated oil. Then it is seasoned differently everyday with different flavorings such as vanilla, cinnamon or various fruits such as banana, apple, lemon, orange juice, or berries.

Use various fruits such as fresh berries, apple, cherry, orange, banana, papaya, grapes etc. Add other fresh fruit if you like, totaling ½ to 1 cup of fruit. Budwig specially advised to use berries like strawberry, blueberry, raspberry, cheery 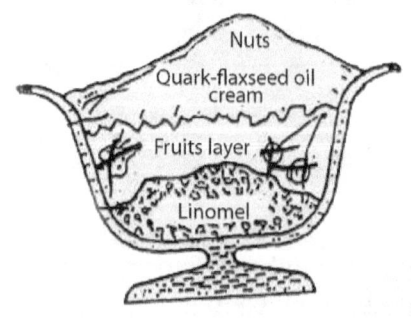 etc. because berries have ellagic acids which are strong cancer fighters.

Add organic raw nuts such as walnuts, almonds, raisins or Brazil nuts. They have sulfurated proteins, omega-3 fats and vitamins. Brazil nut is especially important because a single nut provides you with all of the selenium you need for the day. Selenium is very important to boost immune power. Peanuts are prohibited.

For variety and flavor, try natural vanilla, cinnamon, lemon juice, pure cocoa or shredded coconut.

Once blended in Budwig Cream, Quark and Flax seed oil form a new substance called lipoprotein. Lipoprotein is a water soluble complex. The Quark is rich in the sulfur-containing amino acids, methionine and cysteine. These positively charged amino acids attract the negatively charged electron clouds in fatty acid chains and exhibit a stabilizing effect on the highly unsaturated, otherwise easily oxidized fats. Thus, the amino acids protect the polyunsaturated fatty acids from the Flax seed oil against oxidation which, as a result, are able to enter the human body unchanged and with their full energy potential. The result: they are much more valuable to cells and their membranes. Consequently, one could say that Quark excels as a protector for the polyunsaturated fatty acids.

Sulfur-rich amino acids play a wealth of roles in many vital functions in our bodies. In combination with polyunsaturated fatty acids, they are important partners in regulating the uptake of oxygen and its utilization by the cell. They therefore contribute significantly to a strong immune system, healthy metabolism, and mental vitality. For many generations, people have been getting their omega-3 fatty acids from fish, vegetables, nuts, and seeds. Our health literally depends on the regular consumption of the essential omega-3 and omega-6 fatty acids, alpha-linolenic acid (ALA) and linoleic acid (LA). Our bodies require these fatty acids in order to synthesize their cell membranes as well as for a variety of metabolic processes and heal the cancer and other diseases.

Tips for making the Budwig Mixture

- Follow directions properly! It is important to add things to the mixture in the right order. If you mix them in the wrong order you may lose a lot of the opportunity to convert the oil-soluble omega-3 into water soluble-omega-3.

- Keep the Flax seed oil refrigerated.
- Immersion blender is a must.
- The mixture can be flavored differently every day by adding nuts and fruits preferably organic such as pecans, almonds or walnuts (not peanuts), banana, organic cocoa, shredded coconut, pineapple (fresh) blueberries, raspberries, cinnamon, vanilla or (freshly) squeezed fruit juice.
- Consume immediately for best results.

10 AM Vegetable juice

Freshly squeezed vegetable juice from carrots, beets, celery, tomato, and radish, lemon as well as green vegetables - stinging nettle, lettuce or spinach. Apple is added to sweeten and enhance the taste. Carrot & beet juices are especially helpful to the liver and have strong cancer fighting properties. Vary vegetables. Some tasty and nutritious combinations are beet and apple juice, carrot and apple, carrot and beet, asparagus and apple, celery and apple, celery and carrot. Beet juice should not be taken alone. If taken alone it may cause red or pink urine (beeturia).

She also frequently recommended the following juices:

1. Nettle juice - Especially in the spring, Dr Budwig recommended to puree nettles with water and a lemon.

2. Radish juice - For this, a radish is first crushed and then thrown together with a lemon into the juicer. This juice is by the way durable for several days and Dr Budwig has sometimes recommended her patients to drink a small quantity of them every day.

3. Coltsfoot juice - For this juice, with the exception of the harder old rootstock, the entire remaining underground shoot is mixed with a few flowers and some milk and honey.

4. Horseradish juice - Mix 3-5 cm horseradish together with an apple and (raw) milk. Depending on the quantity of milk you can change the taste. Dr Budwig recommended this juice above all to workmen and to stimulate the appetite. Freshly pressed means, by the way, that you drink the juice within 5 minutes after pressing. In some cases, Dr Budwig prescribed a second juice 30 to 60 minutes later.

12:15 PM Lunch

Salad Platter: Salad plate with homemade cottage cheese-Flax seed mayonnaise. As salad also use: dandelion, cress, celery, tomato, cucumber, lettuce, radish, cabbage, broccoli, green horseradish and pepper.

Delicious mayo salad dressing can be prepared by mixing together 2 Tbsp (30 ml) Flax Oil, 2 Tbsp (30 ml) milk, and 2 Tbsp (30 ml) cottage cheese. Then add 2 tablespoons (30 ml) of Lemon juice (or Apple Cider Vinegar) and add 1 teaspoon (2.5 g) Mustard powder plus some herbs of your choice. Other alternative dressing can be made by mixing Flax Oil, lemon juice, Mustard and some herbs (Budwig, The Oil-Protein Diet Cookbook, 1994).

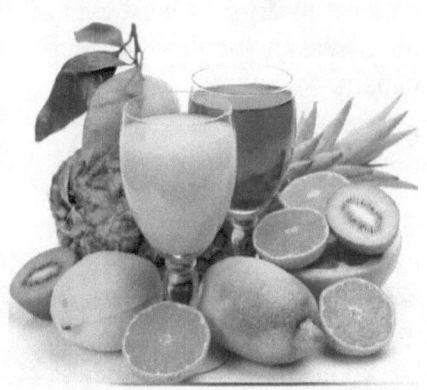

Main Course: Vegetables cooked in water, then flavored with Oleolox and herbs possibly with oatmeal, soy sauce, curry etc. Vegetable broth flavored with a little Oleolox and yeast flakes. As side dish for the vegetables: buckwheat, brown rice, millet or potatoes can be used. One or two slices of Ezekiel bread can be taken. Use lot of dried fruits in the main meal also.

Lunch Dessert: Cottage cheese/ Flax oil mixture served as a dessert, prepared with dry fruits and fruits such as apple, or poured over a fruit salad. You already know how to prepare it perfectly. You will find wonderful recipes for a delicious dessert in the Oil-Protein cookbook by Budwig. Please note that the dessert is **"a must"** and should definitely be eaten. So keep your main course light so you may enjoy the dessert happily.

The form of preparation as "fruit foam," "Linovita" or "red coat in the snow" (in Oil-Protein cookbook) is always welcoming for the healthy and the sick. In all the gimmicks in the preparation of the delicious desserts, one should be aware: Quark and Flaxseed give the patient immense power within a short space of time. Always fresh and beautiful, always freshly interesting, this important food for life should be for the sick and for the whole family.

3 PM Fruit juices

In the afternoon, Dr Budwig recommended different kinds of fruit juices e.g. apples, grapes, cherries, pineapples, papaya, or apricot, sparkling wine or wine - with or without Flaxseeds or with or without a few drops Flaxseed oil.

Budwig preferred papaya juice and recommended her patients to drink at least every 2 days a glass of papaya juice. The main reason for this was definitely the protein splitting enzyme papain.

6 PM Dinner

The evening meal should be light and served early, around 6 p.m. A warm meal may be prepared using brown rice, buckwheat or oat meal. Never consume corn or soy beans. Dishes made with buckwheat grouts are most easily tolerated and nourishing. Use only honey to sweeten. Soup or more solid dishes can be combined with a tasty sauce according to preference. Use OLEOLOX liberally also to sweet sauces and soups, making them nourishing and a richer source of energy.

8:30 PM

A glass of organic red wine may be consumed. All things are a matter of correct dosage. This glass of red wine is not a "must" program. In fact, seriously ill patients having pain and discomfort just starting on the oil-protein diet, it is recommended to serve a glass of red wine mixed with freshly ground Flax seeds to tide them over while going off pain killers (Budwig, Cancer The Problem And The Solution).

METRIC CONVERSION TABLE	
10 g = 0.35 oz	5 cc = 1 teaspoon
100 g = 3.5 oz	15 cc = 1 tablespoon
150 g = 5.25 oz	30 cc = 1 ounce
250 g = 8.8 oz	250 cc = 1 cup
454 g = 1 lb	960 cc = 1 qt
Oz = ounce lb = pound qt = quart Tsp = teaspoon Tbsp = tablespoon	

Precautions

Drink filtered water - Use RO (Reverse Osmosis)water for drinking, cooking and enemas.

Eat Organic Diet - Always try to eat organic food.

Dental Care –

Mercury is a Carcinogenic as well as a Poison! The root canals of dead teeth are full of bacteria that attack the liver and lymphatic system. From Amalgam fillings the mercury slowly leaks out of the filings. The ADA cleverly defends the use of amalgam in spite of the fact that there is sufficient evidence that patients with many severe problems, including psychotic episodes and fatal allergic reactions, were just cured by removing the amalgam. It is advisable to rather have a ceramic filling than be slowly poisoned by mercury. Even gold filling is dangerous; it

135

acts as battery producing electrical current. Be informed that the effect of drugs, including poison, is dose dependant and cumulative.

Fluoride is not only toxic but it is also carcinogenic. Fluoride has never been proven to prevent tooth decay. It has been outlawed in many countries or groups of countries because the evidence is overwhelming that fluoride causes premature aging, so drink bottled water and use fluoride-free toothpaste (American Cancer Institute - 1963).

I highly recommend helping you avoid fillings in the first place. Holistic dentist recommend 3% H_2O_2 as a gargle or rinse, or making a paste using baking soda. H_2O_2 usage three times a day is advised. It is great for cleaning dentures, too.

Frying and deep frying - Frying and deep frying is not allowed to cook patient's food. Never heat any oil in the kitchen. By heating oils the wealth of high energy electrons is destroyed and Trans fats and dangerous toxic chemicals such as acrylamides are formed in the oil.

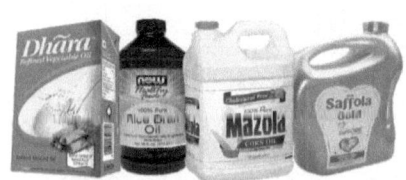

Boiling and steaming are good practices. You can fry vegetables etc. in water and add oleolox before serving. Water is the safest medium for frying, says Lothar Hirneise.

Chemo and Radio -

Chemotherapy is aimed at destruction of the tumor, and it destroys many living cells, and

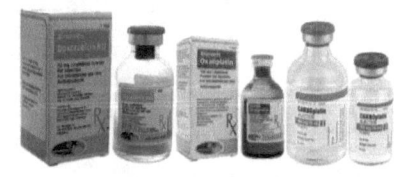

the entire person. Anything that disturbs growth is fatal because growth is an elementary function of life. We cannot achieve something good with bad tools.

Dr. Budwig rejects Chemo and Radiation Therapy. Budwig used to say with full confidence and clarity, "My treatment targets on the real cause of cancer; it fills cancer cells with high

136

energy pi-electrons and attracts oxygen into the cells. And cancer cells start to breathe and produce vital energy."

Man-made Supplements - With this treatment man-made antioxidants, synthetic vitamins and pain killers should not be given. The dose of anticoagulants and aspirin should be adjusted by your doctor. Dr. Budwig favors natural, herbal and homeopathy instead of man-made and synthetic supplements, vitamins and pain killers (Budwig, Cancer The Problem And The Solution).

Prohibitions of Budwig Protocol

In this protocol there are certain restrictions. They are as important as the diet itself. It is very difficult to defeat the cancer without strictly following these rules.

Sugar is strictly forbidden

Sugar, Jiggery, molasses, maple syrup and artificial sweeteners like xylitol, aspartame are not permitted. You can use only natural honey, stevia and fruit juices – all off course unprocessed.

Avoid meats, eggs and fish

Meat, fish, poultry, eggs, and butter are never allowed. Preserved meat is like a poison. It is highly processed and treated with dangerous antibiotics, preservatives and nitrates.

Stop using Hydrogenated Fat and Refined oil

You can never eat pizza, burger, fast food, fried food, biscuits etc. as they all are made by hydrogenated margarine and shortenings. Hydrogenation is a very dangerous process, used to increase shelf life of fats. In this process (oil is heated at very high temperature and hydrogen is passed through oils in presence of nickel) killing Trans fats are formed, high energy live and vital electrons are destroyed and nutrients are damaged. Hydrogenated Fats is just a dead, nutrition-less and cancer causing liquid plastic. Budwig always preached against these damaging fats. She has allowed low fat cheese, oleolox and coconut oil.

Preservatives and Processed Food

You should not eat Potato chips, soft drinks etc. which are full of preservatives. Never consume highly processed food e.g. ready to eat packed foods, pasta, pastries, bread and soy products, tofu etc. However good quality soy souse is permitted.

Microwave, Teflon, Aluminum and Plastic

Never cook in microwave oven. Food cooked in microwave become toxic and deformed. Also don't use aluminum, plastic, Teflon coated cookware and aluminum foils. Use stainless steel, iron, china clay or glass utensils instead.

Chemicals and pesticides are not allowed

Avoid pesticides and chemicals, even those in household products & cosmetics. Stay away from mosquito repellants, sun screen lotions and sun glasses.

Wear natural fibers

Don't wear clothes made using synthetic fiber like nylon, polyester and acrylic. Budwig put great emphasis on the fact that her patients only wore natural fabrics such as cotton or satin, since they too can influence the magnetic field of our body.

Bed

Don't use on foam pillow and mattress. She recommended horsehair mattresses. Latex mattresses are the second choice. In any case, however, you should always replace mattresses that have metal spring cores.

CRT TV and mobile phones

These emit dangerous electromagnetic radiation, so do not use them. You can watch LCD and plasma TVs.

No left over

Food should be prepared fresh and eaten soon after preparation to maximize intake of health giving electrons and enzymes (Budwig, Cancer The Problem And The Solution).

Few Desserts recipes by Dr. Budwig

Fujiya delight

Ingredients for 3 people:
> 250 cc grape juice, 250 cc pure currant juice,
> 8g agar-agar, Quark-Flaxseed oil,
> Milk, honey, vanilla cream

Preparation:

Heat the grape juice till it boils, then add the currant juice, agar-agar, stirring constantly for 5 minutes, and allow to cool. Now divide this mass to 3 narrow, tall cups, which have been rinsed with cold water. It is preferable if these cups have a bottom diameter of only 3- 4 cm. Refrigerate to cool. Now mix a Quark-Flaxseed oil cream with milk, honey and vanilla. Turn the red jelly upside down onto glass plates. The Quark-Flaxseed oil cream is placed on the top so that only the upper half is covered with the Quark-Flaxseed oil cream, so that top looks like the Snow caped Mount Fujiyama.

(The beautiful hotel with a gorgeous view of the Fujiyama is called "Fujiya", hence the dessert "Fujiya".)

Linovita-in-love in wine jelly

Ingredients: for 5 people:
> 250 cc of grape juice, 250 ccm of white wine,
> 8 agar-agar, 4 tablespoons of milk,
> 8 tablespoons of Flaxseed oil, 2 teaspoons of honey,
> 200-250 g of Quark, 2 liqueur glasses
> Vodka, plum (Slibowitz) or cherry brandy or rum

Preparation:

The wine jelly is prepared by heating 250 cc of grape juice till it boils. Agar-agar is stirred with a little wine and placed in the boiling grape juice. Immediately remove from the cooking plate and add the remaining wine gradually with constant stirring.

After about 5 minutes, the jelly mixture clears itself. You can now divide to approx. 5 glass bowls or champagne glasses. Immediately afterwards, mix the Quark-Flaxseed oil cream from Flaxseed oil, milk, honey and Quark. Finally, add 2 liqueur glasses of vodka or slibovitz or cherry brandy or rum into the Quark-Flaxseed oil cream. This Quark-Flaxseed oil mixture is evenly divided on the ready to-use bowls so that the Quark-Flaxseed oil cream partly sinks down in the middle. It is served after complete solidification.

Ice cream with cocoa

Ingredients:
   3 tablespoons of Flaxseed oil, 3 tablespoons of milk,
   1 tablespoon of honey, 100g of Quark, 100 g of hazelnuts,
   2 tablespoons of cocoa

Preparation:
   Quark, Flaxseed oil, milk and honey are mixed in the blender, then the hazelnuts are added, well blended and finally, cocoa is added to the mixture. Now pour the entire mixture into the ice-maker and place it in the fridge compartment of the refrigerator. This mixture with a nougat flavor gives the various combinations mentioned here the dark color contrasts. For very ill people these preparations are very important, especially when there is a general lack of appetite.

*(*Oil-Protein Diet by Lothar Hirneise *available at*
http://www.hirneise.com/page-8/page-19/)

140

ELDI oils

Dr. Budwig created unique ELDI oils, called electron differential oils after performing precise spectroscopic measurements of the light absorption in different oils - specifying that the oils contained pi-electron clouds from Flax oil, wheat germ oil plus vitamin-E in its natural complex, etheric oils and sulfhydryl groups.

Dr. Johanna Budwig said, "The sun is my preferred treatment modality, as is ELDI oil, used externally to stimulate the absorption of the long-wave band of the sun. I have used ELDI oils extensively since 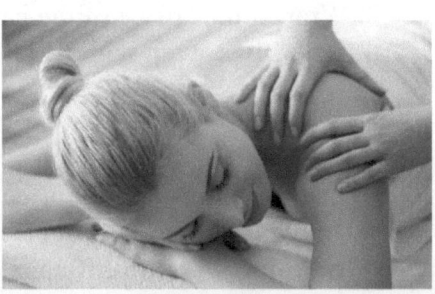 1968 for body massage as well as in the selective application of oil packs. US pain institute has written somewhere: "What this crazy woman does with her ELDI oils, none of us manages to do via pain killers." Dr. Budwig has mentioned that if ELDI oil is not available, you may use Flax oil instead. *You can buy ELDI oils at: www.sensei.de*

Massage Benefits

- Since ancient time massage has been part of cancer healing. Think of your lymphatics as a trash-disposal system for your body. Massage initiates lymphatic drainage, you push the trash out of your body and you're helping your immune system.
- Massage therapy is sometimes the first really pleasant touch a patient is able to experience.
- Massage also releases endorphins (our body's natural painkillers), stimulates lymph movement, and stretches tissues throughout the body. It's energizing, stimulating, and pretty good feeling.

141

ELDI oil plans:

A: For cancer patients in support of the energy level

1. Full-body rubbings in the morning
2. ELDI oil R enema with 200ml every 2-3 days
3. Wrap at the "place of the happening"

B: For energetically weak patients

1. Full-body rubbings in the morning and in the evening
2. Enema: standard plan for ELDI oil R
3. Wrap at the "place of the happening"
4. Daily liver wrap with ELDI oil sage

Additional information:

- Make sure that you make once a week an (deep/high) enema with water or coffee.
- If you make daily coffee enemas, then start in the morning with the coffee enema and then with the ELDI R enema, but only if your energetic level allows you to make two enemas daily. Otherwise, only make the ELDI R enema. (Oil Protein Diet by Lothar Hirneise)

ELDI oils from SENSEI (www.sensei.de) are produced in a permanent cold chain in a European oil mill and marketed under the name of Electron Differentiation Oils. There are two qualities. A 6-star organic quality and a 5-star quality, which are produced exclusively for the IOPDF (www.iopdf.com).

Cost factor ELDI oils

Again and again we hear that for reasons of cost, patients use Flax seed oil instead of ELDI oil R for an enema. Please do not do so, because Flax seed oil does not react in the same way as ELDI oil R. Instead, use cheap ELDI oils from IOPDF or reduce the amount of oil.

Procedure –

Two times a day, i.e. morning and evening, rub ELDI Oil or Flax oil into the skin over the whole body, a bit more intensely on the shoulders, armpits and groin area (where plenty of lymphatic vessels are present) as well as the problem areas, such as the breast, stomach, liver, etc. Leave the oil on the skin for about 20 minutes and follow with a warm water shower without washing with soap. After 10 minutes take another shower, this time using a mild soap, and then relax for 15-20 minutes.

Once the body has been oiled and the ELDI Oil or Flax oil has penetrated the skin, the warm water will open the skin pores and the oil penetrates the skin more deeply. The second shower, where one washes with soap, cleanses the skin so that clothes and linen will not become overly soiled.

Oil Packs

Take a piece of cloth made of pure cotton. Cut to a size to fit the body part, such as the knee. Soak the cotton cloth with oil, place on the knee etc., cover it with a piece of polythene and wrap it up with an elastic bandage. Leave overnight. Remove in the morning and wash the knee; repeat in the evening. Keep applying the same procedure for weeks, you get good results. You also use Flax oil or castor oil for these local applications if you do not get ELDI oils . Dr Budwig generally recommended ELDI sage and should be used in the following indications:

- Tumors
- Painful skin areas
- Metastases
- Hepatic impairment and liver support
- Kidney problems
- Bladder disorders
- Intestinal cramps
- Lung disorders
- Bone disorders of all kinds

ELDI Oil Enema

Enemas are used in the Oil-Protein Diet exclusively for the energy intake and not for the purification of the intestine. Dr Budwig used to give ELDI oil or Flax oil enema to her serious patients. Budwig used to get immediate and miraculous results with the most seriously ill patients. Flax seed Oil enema also give similar results.

I recommend you to make the first enemas only with 100ml and then increase over several days to 250ml. Some patients have enemas with 500ml oil and positively reported on it. 500ml are however the absolute exception and mostly not necessary. Usually 250ml suffice.

Incidentally, smaller amounts are also easily introduced with an enema syringe instead of with an enema bucket. Enema syringes are available in sizes up to 350ml and are easy to handle.

Standard plan for ELDI oil R: Day 1 = 100ml, day 2 = 100ml, day 3 = 150ml, day 4 = 150ml, day 5 = 200ml, day 6 = 200ml and day 7 = 250ml.

From the seventh day, one remains at 250ml, and so long until the patient is significantly better. Then you can go back to 100ml - 150ml, always together with 1-2 daily whole body rubbings. (Oil Protein Diet by Lothar Hirneise)

Ingredients

- Enema pot
- Watch
- A bowl to collect oil when you are getting rid of bubbles.
- Towel and tissue
- RO filtered water
- ELDI oil or Flax oil
- Towel or Drip Stand

Procedure

Prepare a place near the toilet, so that if you can't hold the enema, you will be making a quick dash and the shorter distance is better.

Cleansing Enema with Plain water

First of all you should take a plain water enema. Purpose of this enema is cleaning of intestines. It is not a retention enema

144

and is evacuated immediately. For this you may use 500-1000ml (2-4 cups) RO filtered water. As soon as the whole water is inside the rectum, go and sit on the commode and release the water slowly.

Take the oil enema immediately after the water enema

- Use advised (above) amount of ELDI or Flax oil. The oil should be at body temperature. The best test is to dip your little finger into the oil.
- Fill the oil into the enema pot. It takes at least 5 minutes for the bubbles to get out of the tube.
- The enema pot should be hanged on a drip stand about 2-3 feet above your body.
- You need to lubricate the nozzle and anus with Flax oil. When all is ready, lie on your right side in the fetal position. Insert the nozzle into the rectum slowly and carefully with your left hand, and un-pinch the tube.
- If you feel little uncomfortable when the oil is going in, pinch the tube, wait till the feeling passes away, then continue again.
- The oil is much more viscous and moves more slowly. You might need to hold the pot a bit higher to get it to run a bit quicker.
- Once the oil is in, wait and hold it for about 12 minutes. After that slowly turn yourself to left side and hold oil for another 12 minutes. You may listen to music while taking enema.
- When done, it is best to sit on the commode for about 15 minutes with something to read (Skelton).

Coffee Enema

Dr. Max Gerson introduced coffee enema back in the 1930s. In this enema about 500ml of coffee is pushed into rectum, this amount only reaches up to sigmoid colon. There is no loss of minerals and electrolytes in Coffee Enema because their absorption occurs well before sigmoid colon. Coffee enema is

145

even safe for those who are allergic to coffee because it is not absorbed into the systemic circulation. You may take this enema once or twice. It has the following benefits:

- **Powerful and Natural Pain Reliever**
- **Cleansing** - Coffee also acts as an astringent in the large intestine, helps cleanse the colon walls.
- **Toxin Elimination** - The major benefit of the coffee enema is elimination of toxins through the liver. Caffeine, theophylline and theobromine dilate the blood vessels and bile ducts, stimulate the liver to discharge more bile and boost the detoxifying process into high gear and heal inflammation. Indeed, endoscopic studies confirm they increase bile output.
- **Stimulates Liver** - Kahweol and cafestol palmitate found in coffee promote the activity of a key enzyme system called glutathione S-Transferase. This is an important mechanism in the detoxification of carcinogens, as the enzyme group is responsible for neutralizing free radicals. Coffee enema stimulates the activity of this system by 600- 700%.

Coffee Enema Procedure
- This enema is retained for 12-14 minutes, during this time blood circulates in liver three times and blood is purified. Coffee enema can be given several times a day, few patients take up to seven times a day. Normally if pain is not relieved it may be taken more than one time. You should relax while taking enema; you may listen to music or read newspaper while relaxing. The best time for coffee enema is either early morning after you passed motion or during the day time.

146

- Grind organic coffee beans. Put approx. 750ml of filtered water in a steal pan and bring it to boil. Add 2-5 heaped Tbsp coffee powder, 3 Tbsp is ideal. It is roughly 20-25grams. Let it continue to simmer for ten minutes or more and then turn off the burner. Allow it to cool down to a very comfortable, tepid temperature. Test it with your finger. It should be the same temperature as your body's temperature. Filter the coffee with fine mesh steal sieve into a jug. This is approximately 500ml.
- Pour 2 cups (500ml) of coffee into the enema pot. Be sure the plastic hose is clamped tightly. Now open the clamp and grasp, but do not close the clamp on the hose. Place the enema tip in the sink. Hold up the enema bag above the tip until the coffee begins to flow out. As soon as it starts flowing, quickly close the clamp. This expels any air in the tube.
- Lubricate the enema tip with a small amount of coconut oil or KY jelly. Create a comfortable and relaxing atmosphere. After a few days you will thoroughly enjoy this ritual.
- Light a candle, play some light music and most importantly, make sure you are comfortable and warm. We recommend placing a pillow with a washable cover under your head and lying down on an old towel.
- The position preferred is lying on your back. With the clamp closed hang the pot about 3 feet above your belly. We like to hang the enema pot on a drip stand.
- Insert the tip gently into anus and open the clamp slowly. You should relax and breathe. The coffee may take a few seconds to begin flowing. If you develop a cramp, close the hose clamp, turn from side to side and take a few deep breaths. The cramp will usually pass quickly. Usually nothing happens.
- When all the liquid is inside, close the clamp and remove it slowly. Retain the enema for 12- 14 minutes. You may remain lying on the floor.

- After 14 minutes or so, go to the toilet and empty your gut. Take your time. Wash the enema pot and tube thoroughly with soap and water.
- Take more potassium in the form of fruits and vegetable juices if you take coffee enema regularly (S.A.Wilsons.com).

Epsom bath

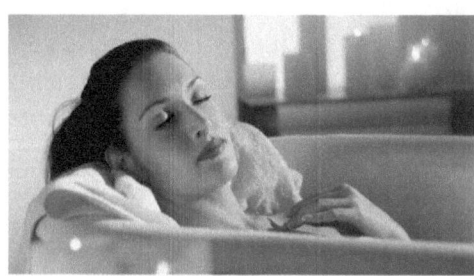

Detoxification of your body through bathing is an ancient remedy that anyone can perform in the comfort of your own home. Your skin is known as the third kidney, and toxins are excreted through sweating. An Epsom salt bath is thought to assist your body in eliminating toxins as well as absorbing the magnesium and nutrients that are in the water. Soaking in Epsom salt actually helps replenish the body's magnesium levels, combating hypertension. The sulfate flushes toxins and helps form proteins in brain tissue and joints. Most of all, it will leave you relaxed, refreshed and awakened. Take it once a week or as advised.

Prepare your bath

- It is a 40 minutes ritual. The first 20 minutes are said to help your body remove the toxins, while the second 20 minutes are for absorbing the minerals from the water
- Fill your tub with comfortably hot water. Use a chlorine filter if possible.
- Add Epsom salt (Magnesium sulfate). For people 50 Kg and up, add 2 cups or more to a standard bath tub.
- Then add 2 cups or more of soda bicarb. It is known for its cleansing ability and even has anti-fungal properties. It also leaves skin very soft.

148

- Add 2-3 Tbsp ground ginger. While this step is optional, ginger can increase your heat levels, helping to sweat out more toxins. However, since it is heating the body, it may cause your skin to turn slightly red for a few minutes, so be careful with the amount you add. Depending on the capacity of your tub, anywhere from 1 Tbsp to 1/3 cup can be added (Herneise).
- Add aromatherapy oils. Again optional, but there are many oils that will make the bath an even more pleasant and relaxing experience (such as lavender), as well as those that will assist in the detoxification process (tea tree or eucalyptus oil). Around 20 drops is sufficient for a standard bath.
- Swish all of the ingredients around in the tub, and then slip into the tub. You should start sweating within the first few minutes. If you feel too hot, start adding cold water into the tub until you cool off.
- Get out of the tub slowly and carefully. Your body has been working hard and you may get lightheaded or feel weak and drained. On top of that, the salts make your tub slippery, so stand with care.
- Drink plenty of water and relax in bed for a few minutes

Soda bicarb bath

Lothar Hirneise has given lot of importance to Soda bicarb bath. It is thought to assist you in eliminating toxins as well as making your body alkaline so your tumor cells may suffocate. Patient may take it once or even twice a day. Just add 2 cups of soda bicarb in your bath tub filled with warm water and relax in it for 30-40 minutes (Hirneise, 2005).

Sun Therapy

Getting an adequate amount of sunshine is a critical part of Budwig protocol. Once the body has acquired the right oil-protein balance with the Cottage Cheeseand Flax oil, the body develops better capacity to absorb the healing photons from the sun. Remember that for healing of cancer high energy photons from the sun are very important. The sunshine is important to maintain adequate vitamin-D levels in our body. Vitamin-D is a powerful antioxidant that has been linked to preventing many diseases including cancer.

Dr. Budwig's focus was on the importance of photons from the sunbeams and their interaction with vital essential fats (linoleic and linolenic acid) in our body. It is the interaction of photons from the sun and the electrons in proper food that provide the synergistic effect on healing our body. Eating the electron rich Flax oil/Cottage Cheese mixture, must be connected with adequate exposure to sunlight.

There is nothing else on earth with a higher concentration of photons of the sun's energy than man. This concentration of the sun's energy is very much energetic point for humans, with their wave eminently suitable lengths - is improved when we eat electron rich essential oils, which in turn absorbs the photons in the form of electro-magnetic waves of sunbeams.

When you eat the FO/CC mixture, your body becomes a better antenna for the photons from the sunbeam. Your body develops a better ability to absorb the energy from the sun and Transfer it to your cells to perform their vital functions. You become energized at a deep level, and when this happens cancer is healed itself.

It is red light that penetrates deeper in the tissues. In 1968 Dr. Budwig used 695 nm ruby (red) lasers light with success to radiate healthy surrounding cancer tissues in cancer patients.

Oil-Protein Diet while travelling

- In her Oil-Protein Diet Cookbook, Dr. Budwig writes: "While traveling, you can always care for yourself with Linomel and hot or cold milk, and/or fruit juices."

- If you are eating a salad in a restaurant, never take the finished dressings, but use olive oil and vinegar. The chance not to take Trans fats is at the least.
- If you want something to be fried, ask the cook to put it in coconut fat or butter. Butter is present in every kitchen.
- Budwig also recommends eating various types of fresh fish to replace the Flax oil and Quark when travelling. You can protect yourself against harm while travelling by ordering fresh fish such as trout, pike, carp and other fresh fish. However, canned (tinned) fish, also shrimps, prawn and other items which frequently contain artificial coloring agents and harmful chemical preservatives, must be strictly avoided.
- Do not eat the "muesli" in hotels. They are mostly denatured carbohydrates.
- Do not use polyunsaturated oils (Flax seed oil, Oil, pumpkin seed oil, etc.) which are kept at room temperature and all contain Trans fatty acids.

For a long vacation

During your long stay travelling away from home, it is really simple to keep up with the Budwig diet, all that is needed was a little bit of preplanning. You may have a fridge and electric tea kettle in the hotel room, or you carry an ice chest.

Wash all fruits and veggies and make enough juice for the travel day and one more day. You should carry a bowl, fork, spoon, sharp knife, and hand blender, nuts, oatmeal and tea. You carry Flax oil, cottage cheese, fruits and veggies in ice chests for travel.

If you have "eaten something", especially too many carbohydrates in the form of potatoes, rice, noodles or even a "not so healthy dessert/cake", then you should take a walk immediately after eating. (Healing Cancer Naturally)

Making Quark

Quark is a very popular and delicious cheese in Germany. You may find many recipes of making Quark on Google. I am giving you a simple recipe here. In this recipe you will learn how it is easy to make your own homemade Quark.

Ingredients

- 1 liter milk preferably <2% fat
- 500ml cultured buttermilk
- Cheese cloth

Instructions

- In a large glass bowl add milk and buttermilk. Stir well and cover with a clean kitchen towel.
- Let this sit at room temperature for 24 hours. The mixture will thicken slightly.
- Heat the oven to 125^0 F and shut off. Set the bowl uncovered into the oven for about 45 min. The mixture will change to yogurt like texture.
- Add a Cheese cloth to a colander and set on a large bowl.
- Pour the milk mixture into the colander, twist the ends and let drain for about 1 ½ to 2 hours.
- The Quark will be in the towel and the whey will be in the bowl. One liter milk usually yields 200gms of Quark.

Making Cottage Cheese

In some places good quality Cottage Cheese is also not available and you need to make your own. Today I am giving you a very good recipe for home made cottage cheese.

Ingredients

- 1 liter natural, low-fat cow's milk preferably <2% fat
- 1/3 cup Vinegar
- Cold water

Instructions

- Mix 1/3 cup of vinegar in 2 cups of water and keep aside. Diluted vinegar yields soft cheese. You may also use diluted lemon juice.
- Boil the milk in a heavy bottomed pan over medium heat, stirring frequently making sure milk does not burn on the bottom of the pan. As the milk comes to a boil, remove the pan from the gas burner and place it on kitchen counter.
- Now add about a glass of cold water to bring the milk's temperature down to about 75-80 degrees Celsius. We want to curdle the milk at this temperature, so we get a soft cheese.
- Then add little (about 1-2 Tbsp) diluted vinegar slowly and stir the milk gently. After 10 seconds, add little vinegar slowly and stir the milk. Go on adding vinegar until the curd will start separating from the whey. Remember you should curdle the milk slowly.
- Once the cheese has completely separated from the whey, add a glass of cold water and drain the whey using a stainless steel strainer.
- Now Transfer the curdled cheese into a suitable container and blend thoroughly with electric hand blender until you get very smooth and thick creamy cheese. If the cheese is dry, add a little milk while blending. This is your home made cottage cheese.

Buckwheat

Dr. Budwig highly recommended buckwheat in her healing diet. Contrary to its name, this seed is not related to wheat. Buckwheat is a gluten free power food!

Buckwheat is supercharged with health-boosting nutrients and phytochemicals, including B-vitamins, magnesium, manganese, phosphorus, zinc, copper, potassium, and selenium. It is also one of the best natural sources of rutin and D-chiro-

Inositol, two phytochemicals that have been associated with a number of interesting health benefits. It is the best source of high-quality, easily digestible proteins. This makes it an excellent meat substitute. What's more, buckwheat grouts (the hulled kernels) are generally well tolerated and rarely cause allergic reactions or other adverse effects in humans. These gluten-free kernels can be served as an alternative to rice or made into delicious buckwheat porridge.

Studies have shown that populations eating diets high in fiber-rich whole grains and seeds, like buckwheat, consistently have lower risk for colon cancer. Research reported at the American Institute for Cancer Research (AICR) International Conference on Food, Nutrition and Cancer, by Rui Hai Liu, M.D., Ph.D., and his colleagues at Cornell University shows that buckwheat, contain many powerful phytonutrients that can fight cancer.

Energy Healing

Mild exercise

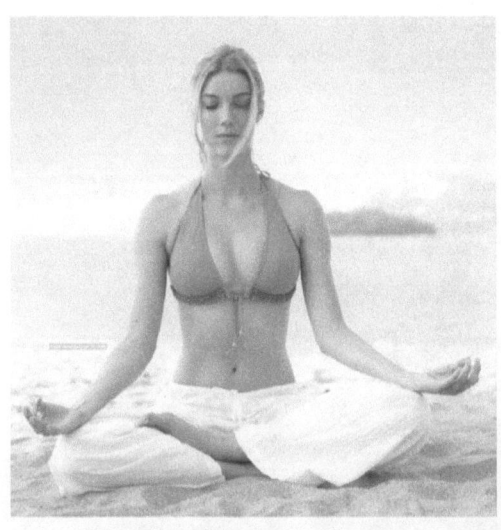

Patient can do mild exercise and remain active if his condition permits. He can go for a walk or do light yoga in the open terrace or garden under the healing and refreshing sunshine. Patient can jog for a few minutes after lunch or dinner. It is very beneficial for cancer patient. But if patient is serious and has metastasis, he should not jog, better he should relax in his house.

Patient can keep himself busy in many activities like sitting in garden enjoying nature, visualization, listening music, reading, laughing, chatting with friends etc. Stress, depression, anxiety, anger and fear can be very damaging to him. Share your feelings with your life partner or a best friend.

You should try your best to remove stress and negative thoughts and balance the flow of energy "prana" or "chi" in your body. Do meditation, Emotional Freedom Technique EFT, Qigong, Reiki, Acupuncture, Acupressure, Sun Salutation etc. to heal your body, mind and spirit.

Meditation

Meditation is a means of transforming the mind. Meditation practices are techniques that encourage and develop concentration, clarity, positivity, and relaxation of the body and mind. Do any simple meditation for relaxation. Meditation stimulates pineal gland (*piyush granthi*) to shower melatonin hormone. Melatonin controls circadian rhythm and induces restorative sleep. Its powerful antioxidant effect offers important enhancements to the brain and nervous system, helping protect against age-related damage. Melatonin is power anti-stress and anticancer hormone.

Yoga Nidra

It is divine sleep with alertness. In 15 minute yoga nidra session, you relax in a fully supported shavasan, limbs limp, breath quiet, thoughts drifting by. In the distance, the 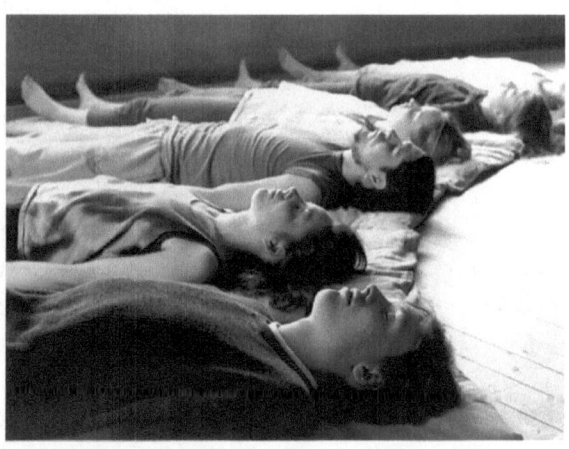 teacher's voice blends with the sound of Tibetan bells. All traces of the day fade away, time stops, and stillness washes over the body. Yoga nidra is a systematic method of complete relaxation, holistically addressing our physiological, neurological, and subconscious needs.

How long should you take this protocol?

If all is well patient feels better and tumor start to shrink within a 3 or 4 months, if he follows treatment religiously and honestly. He may be cured in one or two years. **It is recommended that the Budwig protocol and full diet is followed for at least five years.** Even after that he should maintain healthy eating and life style.

Dr. Budwig has clearly mentioned that if you do not get the desired success, do not blame the protocol, rather try to find out your mistakes and correct them. The threshold between winning and losing is very small, and even a minor mistake can unbalance the complete healing process.

How do I recognize good Flax seed oil?

Good Flax seed oil is unfortunately dependent on many factors. The IOPDF assigns a star for each fulfilled criterion. The best oil has thus 6 stars and the worst gets no star. Let us look at the 6 criteria in detail:

Criterion 1: Cooling chain

Studies have shown that, in addition to processing the Flax seed, cooling is the most important criterion for good Flax seed oil. So buy only Flax seed oil stored in a refrigerated rack and kept in a permanent cold chain. If you shop through the Internet, the Flax seed oil must be delivered in a Styrofoam packaging and as fast as possible.

Criterion 2: Local Flax seed

Weekly shipping on ships and sometimes additional chemicals used can cause great damage to Flax seed. Therefore, make sure that you only buy Flax seed oil whose Flax seed comes from the country where you are living or at least from the same continent. This normally can be seen at the seal.

Criterion 3: Omega-3 fatty acid content

The Oil-Protein Diet is about linolenic acid (omega-3). Buy Flax seed oil with a high amount of linolenic acid. Depending in which country you are living the range can be between 55% - 63%.

Criterion 4: Organic quality

It makes a big difference whether Flax seed grows in biologically controlled soil or in soils of conventional agriculture. So buy only Flax seed oils with organic quality, unless you know the oil mill personally and know what Flax seed the mill is processing.

Criterion 5: glass bottle

Flax seed oil and electron differentiation oils are available in glass and plastic bottles or in canisters, which are mostly made of tinplate. Consumers should only buy oils in glass bottles. Avoid plastic bottles, as they may contain highly toxic softeners.

Criterion 6: Light

Flax seed oil should be packaged and stored in a light-proof package. Therefore, only buy bottles in dark brown or dark green bottles. (Oil Protein Diet by Lothar Hieneise)

Linomel

Linomel is an invention by Dr Budwig. Freshly crushed Flax seed is mixed with honey and milk powder so that the crushed Flax seed is more stable. There is no doubt that freshly crushed Flax seed is more valuable, but also has the disadvantage that you do it yourself and clean the grinder afterwards. That is why Linomel still has an existence right. Do not buy crushed Flax seed in the shop as the chance that these contain Trans fatty acids is 100%.

Is there an alternative to Linomel?
- Freshly crushed Flax seed is an alternative. This must be eaten immediately after the meal, otherwise it will oxidize.
- Make your own Linomel. Mix 6 tablespoons freshly crushed Flax seed with a tablespoon of honey. Small tip: Grind the Flax seed, e.g. in a coffee grinder, and set the grinder to coarse. So it mixes better with the honey.

(Oil Protein Diet by Lothar Hieneise)

Questions and Answers

How do I store Flax seed oil?

Generally cool. Best at 5^0-10^0 (Fahrenheit 41-50) in the refrigerator. Always keep the Flax seed oil bottles upright and never lay them down as they may cause faster oxidation.

Should I now buy low fat Quark or Quark with 20% or 40% fat?

Only a Quark with as little fat (less than 2%) is optimal. Quark is about sulfur-containing amino acids. Less fat means more amino acids.

Can Quark be replaced with tofu, yoghurt or soya?

Absolutely no.

Is there an alternative to Quark?

In many books or on the Internet, it is always claimed that there are alternatives to Quark, such as e.g., yogurt, soy or whey protein (which you should never use!). This is wrong. There is absolutely no good substitute for Quark. The only alternative (although it has a slightly different composition like Quark) is Cottage Cheese with as little fat as possible. This should only be used if no Quark is available.

Can I eat cheese?

Basically yes, but in moderation and with the exception of cream cheese and fresh cheese. Only raw milk/hard cheese is permitted. Cheese of sheep or goat is preferable.

Can I eat raisins and dates?

Yes, raisins and dates are allowed in small quantities.

Which fat can be used for frying?

159

Only coconut fat.

Can I use olive oil?

Theoretically, you can use any organic oils with salad. Dr Budwig preferred Flax seed oil, pumpkin seed oil, wheat germ oil, poppy oil, and thistle oil are also permitted, but do not heat. Oleolox may be heated for two minutes.

Can I drink coffee?

No.

Can soya and oatmeal be eaten?

Dr Budwig wrote several times that oat flakes, soy flakes, yeast flakes and other flakes are permitted. But today I just say that you buy only high quality organic "flakes".

Can I eat bread?

Dr Budwig has recommended her patients to eat no bread during acute tumor phases. Instead, she recommended full-grain rice waffles or Ezekiel bread as an alternative.

Can cows or soy milk be drunk?

No, drinking any milk is forbidden in the Oil-Protein Diet.

Can noodles be eaten?

In the literature of Dr Budwig nearly always did not allow cancer patients to eat noodles. The reason is that noodles are made of flour, eggs and oil. Flour has the disadvantage that it is basically a fast-digesting sugar and mostly the producers use cheap oils. Energetically speaking, noodles are "not really full with electrons". Unfortunately, you are worsening the already bad adrenaline - insulin ratio of a cancer patient.

Which milk can be used for the Quark?

Dr Budwig recommended raw milk. Unfortunately these are nowadays difficult to buy anywhere. Alternatively, pasteurized milk is also okay. All other varieties of milk, such as ultra-heat-treated or homogenized (long life or full cream), are prohibited.

Budwig Diet & Protocol - In Brief

This is raw organic diet with lot of Flax oil and Juices. Consume only clean or RO filtered water. To get the best results, proper guidance is strongly recommended. Below are brief guidelines of the Budwig Diet you don't have to consume all the foods on this list. This information is from Dr. Budwig's books.

First thing in the morning – One glass of sauerkraut juice, preferably raw & homemade. Raw unheated kraut has enzymes, probiotics and vitamins which help the digestive system, metabolize foods & improve immunity.

Just before breakfast - green or herbal tea

Breakfast – First blend 3 Tbsp. Flax oil, 3 Tbsp. milk and a Tsp real honey; then gradually add 6 Tbsp. Quark or Cottage Cheeseand blend. Garnish in layers. Add 2 Tbsp freshly ground Flax seeds n a bowl, then add a layer of crushed fresh fruits, then pour oil cheese mixture and put raw nuts on top. Afterward, if hungry, choose whole grain organic bread, raw vegetables, & quality cheeses such as Edam, Gouda, Emmentaler, Sbrinz or Camembert.

Mid-morning - Homemade vegetable juice (carrots, beets w/lemon or apple, or greens). Homemade carrot or beet juices are very important cancer-fighters.

Before Lunch (especially serious patients) - Champagne with 1 Tbsp ground Flax seeds in small glass of fruit juice. The champagne helps with absorption of the seeds.

Lunch - Salad plate (tomato, cucumber, lettuce, radish, cabbage, broccoli, and pepper) with homemade Cottage Cheeseand Flax oil mayo dressing (prepared by mixing together 2 Tbsp Flax oil, 2 Tbsp milk, 2 Tbsp Cottage Cheeseand 1 Tbsp lemon juice, add a variety of herbs making the plate most appealing.

Lunch - Main Course Vegetables cooked in water, then flavored with oleolox and herbs possibly with oatmeal, curry etc. Vegetable soups flavored with a little oleolox and nutritional yeast flakes, as side dish for buckwheat, brown rice, millet or potatoes.

Lunch Dessert - Must have 2nd serving of 3 Tbsp. Flax oil and 6 Tbsp. Quark or Cottage Cheese with a little milk and honey, well blended. Add raw fruit, fruit juice, raw nuts, and other flavors you like.

Mid-afternoon - 1 Tbsp. freshly ground Flax seed added to 1 glass of pure fruit juice, homemade.

Late afternoon - Papaya or pineapple juice, 1 glass, with 1 Tbsp Flax seeds freshly ground.

Dinner - Grains alone or grains & beans with vegetables with oleolox, nutritional yeast flakes & spices. Eat buckwheat at least 4 days in a week. Grains & beans combined make a complete protein. Vegetables such as spinach, asparagus, broccoli, & cabbage add nutrition and aid absorption. Dine early.

Late Evening - 1 glass red wine (optional). Go to sleep early - before 10 P.M. if possible.

Prohibitions of Budwig Protocol

- No Sugar, no meat, no eggs, no Butter
- No hydrogenated fat and refined oil
- No soya, corn, peanuts and refined table salt
- No frying, no sautéing, no deep frying
- No preservatives and processed Food
- No microwave, Teflon coated and aluminum cookware
- No cosmetics, chemicals and pesticides
- No foam mattress and pillow.
- No nylon, polyester or acrylic clothing, only cotton, silk and wool is allowed.
- No Crt. TV and mobile phones
- No leftover food

Elimination or Detoxification
May include (Remember the Mnemonic - M.Sc. Botany)
- **Flax oil massage,**
- **sun therapy,**
- **coffee enema** and
- **soda bicarb bath,** epsom bath, oil pulling, steam bath, sauna bath, liver, colon and kidney cleansing etc.

Energy Therapies (Remember MTV)

- **Meditation,** Meditation, yoga nidra, positive attitude, system change and deep breathing exercises.
- **Tumor contract** – Tell your tumor that if it grows in size, then you may die, and eventually he also will die. So advise him to become microscopic in size. In return you promise to make some changes in your life so that both of you might live long. If he agrees with your proposal, sign a contract with him immediately.
- **Visualization** – is the most important tool to tap into the power of your imagination to help heal cancer. Remain tuned to your healthy and happy future.

Important and must do therapies with Budwig
- Dandelion root 1 Tsp once or twice a day
- Black seed oil as advised by Maria Hurairah
- Bitter apricot kernels 5 kernels per 5kg of body weight with a Tsp pumpkin seeds
- Essiac tea 30ml to 90ml per day
- Brazil nuts a nut a day
- Nano curcumin 1 cap twice or thrice a day
- and Coenzyme Q-10 1 cap once or twice a day
- Nutritional yeast flakes

Lothar Hirneise

Great supporter of Budwig Protocol

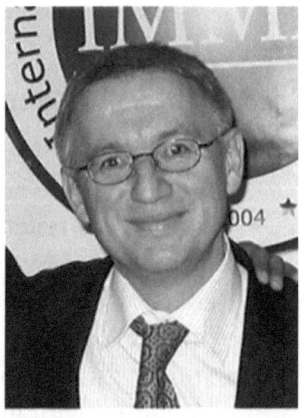

Eleven years, Lothar Hirneise worked as a trained nurse in the State Psychiatric Hospital in Winnenden. After four years, he took psychoanalysis training. Hirneise was also master in Eastern combat sports and a Kung Fu teacher. He owned a successful sporting goods company, which he sold for a tidy profit in 1986. After a year one of his close friend developed Testicular Cancer. Lothar went in search of information about cancer therapies and came across Lynne McTaggart, the founder of the book and magazine "What Doctor's Don't Tell You." Then he was informed that Frank Wiewel, president of the American organization "People Against Cancer", which operates alternative cancer research since 1985, would come to London. So he went to London with his best friend Klaus Pertl to attend this conference for alternative cancer treatments (early 1997). This weekend his friend died. This was the starting point of his intensive quest for potential cancer therapies. He had time and money and read everything he could get his hands on. He nearly went crazy and was severely infected by a virus called Holistic Oncology. He travelled to Bahamas, Mexico, Russia, China, and the United States and all over Europe.

Frank Wiewel advised him to visit Dr. Budwig who lived only 60 km from his home in Germany. Lothar and Klaus Pertl visited Budwig in the spring of 1998, and from the beginning it was an intense relationship that persisted for a very long time.

Over several years he remained in close contact with this great sage of Science. The content of their conversations used to be about fats and electrons. One day she suggested writing a book in which, she could explain her theories again, briefly and concisely. And the Book Cancer - "The Problem And The Solution" was written. Lothar worked very hard in the creation of this great book.

Lothar Hirneise is founder and President of "People Against Cancer", Germany. He is a great researcher and writer on alternative healing. In his book "Chemotherapy cures cancer and the earth is flat" he puts an "Encyclopedia of unconventional cancer treatments", and summarizes the results of his years of worldwide research together. The book became a best seller within no time. He had successfully treated thousands of cancer patients at his center in Germany (3E Zentrum, Buocher Höhe Im Salenhäule 10, D-73630 Remshalden-Buoch Telefon: 07151-98130).

Tumor is not a problem, but a solution

Lothar Hirneise says: "A tumor is the body's solution to some problem in your body. A tumor forms because someone is no longer producing adrenaline, which is needed to break down sugar. An excess of sugar is dangerous, so the body produces tumors. Tumors ferment or burn sugar. Tumors also use a lot of energy - sugar - due to the fast division of cells. Cancer cells function like liver cells, but much more efficiently. So the tumor helps you to get rid of poisons from your body. Without the tumor you would be really ill. That is why you shouldn't immediately operate to remove a tumor. First strengthen and detoxify yourself. If the tumor still continues to grow - which is almost never the case - you can always operate later."

165

3E Program

He travels a lot in search of finding most successful alternative cancer therapies. In the last few years he has interviewed several hundred final stage so-called survivors, meaning patients who were in the final stage of cancer and who are all healthy again today. Based on his findings he proposed a 3E Program for cancer.

- Eat well
- Eliminate the toxins from the body
- Energy

He noticed that 100% of all survivors, did the energy work. In approximately - say 80% of all patients, He found a change in diet. And in at least 60% of all patients, took intensive detoxification rituals. This is the basis of his, so much talked about 3E Program for healing cancer.

Diet and Nutrition

He proudly says that he has shaken the hands with hundreds of people, who made extreme dietary change and became well. They are still alive and living a healthy life. If you still believe that Cancer diets are nonsense, go to him, he will prove the opposite. He has interviewed enough patients and knows them personally. Good nutrition naturally means getting energy. He explains that we have three ways and means of getting energy into our bodies.

1. The first is the light. Light is naturally our number one source of energy. He is 100% sure.

2. The second way is organic nutrition. He emphasized strict organic diet; of course, you do not get any energy from a chicken burger. Rather, when you eat this, you lose some energy, which you have to compensate later.

3. Another possibility which you have is let the energy flow in your body, in your meridians and in your thoughts. Think

about the feeling you had last time when you were in love. You felt wonderful; you were on top of the sky. But what did it change? Did your DNA change? Did your cell respiration change? Nothing really changed. The Indians would say your chakras were opened and the energy started to flow freely again. This is the secret, not only to get the energy, but also to let it flow freely. This proves that our thoughts, our mental-spiritual side is too important.

Now back to nutrition. Out of all nutritional therapies of cancer that he had investigated, the Budwig diet is definitely number one. He investigated thousands of patients, Dr. Budwig allowed him to investigate all her cases of the last thirty years, and he concluded that nowhere you find such fantastic cases as with Dr. Budwig, not even remotely. It's amazing. Even patients who were in coma, when received her Oil-Protein Diet, and rubbed so-called electron differential oils (ELDI oils) on the body, did again come out from coma. They were able to eat, walk and live normally today. It is really miraculous. Therefore, her Oil-Protein Diet became the basis of his 3-E Program for cancer patients.

Detoxification

Next important point that he suggests is detoxification. Detoxification actually covers two points.

1. The first is naturally to avoid toxins and poisons e.g. use of cosmetics, toothpaste, etc.

2. And the second point which belongs to detoxification is not to add any toxins in future. The most important point is definitely diet. It doesn't need further explanation. We are ingesting lot of poisons through our diet. Is better not to eat than all this rubbish that one can buy today.

Healthy teeth and gums are phenomenally important. Heat is a very good way to expel poisons. All the parasite cleanses, colon cleansing, ELDI oils, drinking a lot of water is essential. Going out into the sun light, twice daily is very important. You might

167

have listened today that the sun is suddenly bad for you and may cause skin cancer. That is nonsense, forget it. We are all children of the light, we definitely need the light. Even if it's raining and cloudy today go outside. Even if patient is in coma, he must be wheeled out. You should go twice daily into the light. Light increases Vitamin D levels, important for the liver and increases energy levels.

Energy Work

Energy work is the most important point. He divides it into mental and spiritual work. Naturally, you are advised to do meditation and develop positive thinking. You think about life, 'Why do I have cancer and what is the purpose of my life, why am I here on this earth?' and so on. But he focused on something what he called the **SYSTEM CHANGE**. He explains that we all live in Systems. In our marriage, in our house, in our job, etc. Many, many, many of these cancer patients made system jumps. Means that they kicked their husband in the butt and threw him out. They quit their job, they moved, they not only moved their bed, they moved out of their apartment, went to other countries. Quite honestly, I don't know, what should you do? But Lother's experience is that it it's remarkable to what extent people changed their life before they were in a position to get well.

Lothar Hirneise Concludes: "There is no spontaneous remission, there are only people who positively change their life and regained their health that way." (Hirneise, 2005)

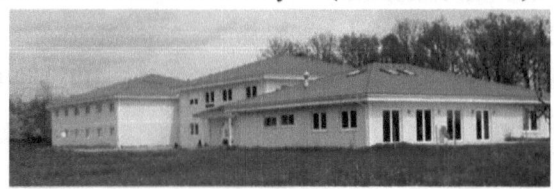

~~**~~

168

Interview of Dr. Johanna Budwig

Lothar Hirneise worked with Dr. Johanna Budwig from 1998 to 2003. He explained that there is much more available to cancer patients than just chemo and irradiation. Mr. Lothar Hirneise conducted this great interview in 1998 (Budwig, Cancer The Problem And The Solution).

Lothar Hirneise: What is your fundamental research?

Dr Johanna Budwig: In 1949, I developed Paper Chromatography of fats with Professor Kaufmann, the director of the Federal Institute for Research on Grain, Potatoes and Fat, and my former doctoral advisor, who was also director of the Pharmaceutical Institute. With this technique for first time I was able to detect fats, fatty acids and lipoproteins directly even in 0.1 ml of blood. I used Co 60 isotopes successfully to produce the first differential reaction for fatty 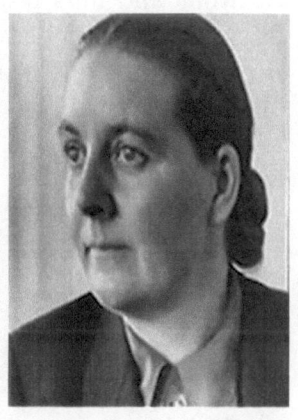 acids, and produced the first direct iodine value via radioiodine. I also developed control of atmosphere in closed system by using gas systems which act as antioxidants. I further developed Coloring, separating effects of fats and fatty acids. I too studied their behavior in blue light, red light with fluorescent dyes.

Using rhodamine red dye, I studied the electrical behavior of the unsaturated fatty acids with their "halo". With this technique I could prove that electron rich highly unsaturated Linoleic and Linolenic fatty acids (Flax oil being richest source) were the mysterious and undiscovered decisive fats in respiratory enzyme function which Otto Warburg could not find. I studied the electromagnetic function of pi-electrons of the linolenic acid in the cell membranes, for all nerve function, secretions, mitosis, as

169

well as cell division. I also examined the synergism of the sulfur containing protein with the Pi-electrons of the highly unsaturated fatty acids and their significance for the formation of the hydrogen bridge between fat and protein, which represent "the only path" for fast and focused Transport of electrons during respiration.

This immediately caused an excitement in scientific community. Everybody thought that it will open new doors in Cancer research. I also proved that Hydrogenated fats, refined oils including all Trans fatty acids were not having any vital electrons and thus proved as respiratory poisons. We published this research exclusively in many journals including "New Directions in Fat Research".

Lothar Hirneise: What is the prime cause of Cancer?

Dr Johanna Budwig: In 1928 Dr. Otto Warburg proved that all normal cells require oxygen absolutely, but cancer cells can live without oxygen. It is a rule without exception. If you deprive a cell 35% of its oxygen for 48 hours and it would become cancerous. Dr. Otto Warburg has proved it clearly that the root cause of cancer is lack of oxygen in the cells, which creates an acidic state in the human body.

He also discovered that cancer cells are anaerobic i.e. do not breathe oxygen, get the energy by fermentation of glucose producing lactic acid and cannot thrive in the presence of high levels of oxygen. Long back in 1911 Swedish scientist Torsten Thunberg postulated that sulfur containing protein (found in cottage cheese) and some unknown fat is required to attract oxygen in the cell. This fat plays a major role in the cellular respiration. For nearly half century scientists were trying to identify this unknown and mysterious fat but nobody succeeded.

Lothar Hirneise: How did you develop cancer therapy which is called Budwig Protocol?

Dr Johanna Budwig: During my research I found that the blood of seriously ill cancer patients had deficiency of unsaturated essential fats (Linoleic and Linolenic fatty acids),

170

lipoproteins, phosphatides, and hemoglobin. I also noticed that cancer patients had a strange greenish-yellow substance in their blood which is not present in the blood of healthy people. I wanted to develop a healing program for cancer.

So I decided to straight way go for human trials and I enrolled 642 cancer patients from four big hospitals in Münster. I started to give Flax oil and Cottage Cheeseto the cancer patients. After just three months, patients began to improve in health and strength, the yellow green substance in their blood began to disappear, tumors gradually receded and at the same time as the nutrients began to rise. Thus I had a cure for cancer. It was a great victory and the first milestone in the battle against cancer. My treatment is based on the consumption of Flax seed oil with low fat cottage cheese, raw organic diet, detoxification, mild exercise, Flax oil massage and the healing powers of the sun. I have treated approx. 2500 cancer patients during last few decades. Prof. Halme of surgery clinic in Helsinki used to keep records of my patients. According to him my success was over 90% and this too was achieved in cases where conventional Oncology failed.

Lothar Hirneise: Can you tell us more about the unsaturated fatty acids and their net-like connections?

Dr. Johanna Budwig: Fatty acid is a carboxylic acid having unbranched chain of 4 to 28 carbons. The saturated fatty acids have primarily short carbon chains. In butter, coconut fat, goat fat and sheep fat the fatty acids consists of 4, 6, 8, 10 or 12 carbons. These fats are saturated, however they can also easily metabolize if the essential fatty acids are present. The unsaturated vital fatty acids really start with the chain with 18 carbon compounds. There are also fatty acids with up to 30 carbons. Fatty acids with 18 carbons, like in Flax oil with the higher level of unsaturation, are more important for human beings, particularly for the brain functions of man. Linoleic acid rich in electrons is considered vital. There is particularly high amount of energy in this double double bonds of the linoleic acid.

171

This energy wanders and is not fixed in place while in a chemical compound, such as with table salt the energy is fixed. This energy, wandering between electrons and the positively charged protein with sulfur groups is an alternating association process in the electromagnetic field. This is very important. Perhaps you are familiar with the painting of Michelangelo, where God creates Adam (two fingers pointing to each other, however they do not touch). This is quantum physics, here the fingers do not touch. The physicists who I know, Max Planck, or Albert Einstein, or Dessauer all represent the view that man is created by God in His image. You see in being together as human beings there is certainly also a connection without directly touching the other person. The dipolarity with a single double bond in olive oil is weaker than it is in sunflower seed oil, which is has two double bonds. This double double bond is considered to be vital for man. However if the same chain length of 18 carbons has three unsaturated fatty acid double bonds, then the electrical energy is as strong as a magnet. This electronic energy is negatively charged. The positively charged sulfur groups of the protein adhere in the unsaturated bonds where the electrons are and that is where they insert their sulfur-containing compounds.

This produces the lipoproteins. The life process is sustained in the interplay between the positively-charged particles and negatively-charged particles. In this process there is no connection, and this is our life element. If radical damage occurs at this point through fatty acids that has lost electron energy, but rather are cross-linked like a net, then the dipolarity can no longer work actively in this net. This is the deadly effect of free radicals, because instead of the chains with the electron clouds they interlace like a net without electron clouds, indeed with unsaturated bonds, but without dipolarity. I quickly knew that the triple unsaturated fatty acids, which were called linolenic acid, and which no one had isolated before me, had 18 carbons and that they did not always carry their double bonds at the same point. They have such a strong electronic energy compared to the heavier matter in the 18-link fatty acid chains, that biologically this energy is far greater than it is with the next arachidonic acid with 20 links. The highest electron collection is with the combination of linoleic-linolenic fatty acids in Flax oil. The linolenic acid as conjugated (interaction of neighboring double bonds in the molecule that are separated by a single bond) fatty acid is even more effective and is even more strongly interplay with linoleic acid as it is present in the Flax oil for oxygen absorption. This was relatively easy for me to verify in my experiments. I would like to emphasize this. The combination of double unsaturated linoleic acid with triple unsaturated linolenic acid is particularly well-combined in Flax seed.

Lothar Hirneise: Is it this energy that heals cancer?

Dr. Johanna Budwig: Yes, this energy is now movable and it is easily released. It is precisely this energy that heals cancer, or does not even allow it to occur. If this vital element is present then no tumor can exist. This vital element is a deciding factor in the immune system. There is no effective factor in the immune system other than the essential fatty acids.

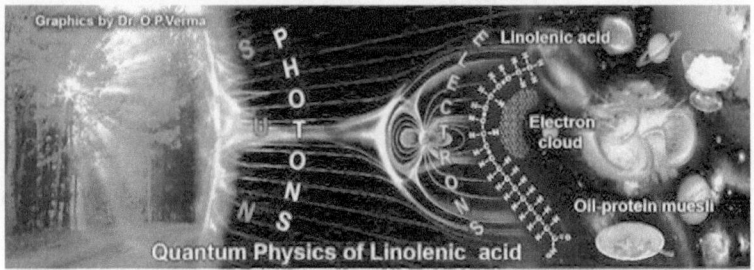

Lothar Hirneise: What is an electron cloud?

Dr Johanna Budwig: If the enhancement of electronic energy is always higher through absorption of sun photons in the unsaturated fatty acids e.g. in linolenic fatty acids, then the power of the electrons is so high in the dipolarity between gravity and electrons, that they lifts off of the heavy mass and floats like a cloud hence I called them electron cloud.

Lothar Hirneise: What is the significance of the cloud?

Dr. Johanna Budwig: No life form has as much energy to store the electrons and photons as doe's man. The electronic

173

energy stored particularly in the vital, highly unsaturated fatty acids, is very strong life element for man. Man cannot live without them. If oils are treated with heat and harsh chemicals (during refining and hydrogenation process to increase their shelf life) then the wealth of vital electronic energy is destroyed and Trans fats are formed with net like connections. They are no longer vital fats with 18 carbons, but rather they form cross-links between the fatty acids like a large net, and are highly damaging to our body, do not adhere with proteins, do not attract oxygen and act like a free radicals. I repeat because it is so important: I have detected particles in oils treated with steam, which indeed have a positive iodine value, but which are highly toxic for man.

Lothar Hirneise: So you preach against these toxic hydrogenated and refined oils?

$$-\underset{\underset{\text{H}}{|}}{\overset{\overset{\text{H}}{|}}{\text{C}}}-\underset{\underset{\text{H}}{|}}{\overset{\overset{\text{H}}{|}}{\text{C}}}- \qquad -\overset{\overset{\text{H}}{|}}{\text{C}}=\overset{\overset{\text{H}}{|}}{\text{C}}- \qquad -\overset{\overset{\text{H}}{|}}{\text{C}}=\underset{\underset{\text{H}}{|}}{\text{C}}-$$

Saturated Fat	Unsaturated Fat	Trans fat

Dr. Johanna Budwig: I am completely against using these "pseudo" fats - "hydrogenated" or "partially hydrogenated". These are the biggest enemy of mankind. I had scientific proofs. The heart rejects these fats and they are deposited as inorganic fat on the heart muscle itself. They end up blocking circulation, damage heart action, inhibit cell renewal and impede the free flow of blood and lymph fluids.

But it was highly profitable business for multinationals. When I preached against these fats, they stood against me, first they tried to bribe me and when I refused they filed many fake court cases against me. I was working for humanity and had scientific proof. I was like rock of Gibraltar in my decision; I fought and won all the cases ultimately.

174

Lothar Hirneise: What is your view point about surgery for tumors?

Dr. Johanna Budwig: I am totally against radiation and chemo; I also reject hormonal treatment. Surgery must be considered individually. I am not a proponent of quickly making artificial anus. Conventional oncology no longer does justice to the cancer patients.

Lothar Hirneise: You also studied medicine at the age of 47 years.

Dr. Johanna Budwig: (smiling) Yes handsome! That's right, my opponents were accusing me that how can I treat cancer patients without a doctors degree. This thing pinched me, so in 1955, I joined medical school in Göttingen. There I was using my therapy very successfully in various clinics. I still remember the time I was working late one night in Göttingen, a woman came to me, with her small child whose arm was supposed to be amputated due to a tumor. I treated her and soon the subject of amputation was dismissed and the child quickly did very well.

Because I was still a medical student at this time, I was summoned to appear before the Municipal Court due to a petition that I should be prohibited from studying medicine. I explained the truth in the court. The judge rejected the case and said, "You have done a good job, Budwig. In my area of jurisdiction nothing will happen to you. If it does there will be a scandal in the scientific community."

Lothar Hirneise: What do you recommend for prevention of cancer?

Dr. Johanna Budwig: Consume only Flax oil as oil. I reject frozen and preserved meat. Fresh meat is OK. No frozen food and no bakery products. Avoid all Trans fats. Eat organic diet. Oleolox should be used as butter. Prepare fruit juices yourself. Cheese and potatoes are OK. Also the electromagnetic environment (e.g. microwave and mobile phones etc.) in which we live is very important. I reject synthetic textiles and foam

175

mattresses because they steal lot of electrons from you. A lot of wood in home construction and woolen or silk carpets are also important. Wear gemstones, they also have good biological radiation. Books could be written on gemstones. The environment and living conditions must be as biological (organic & natural) as possible. Regular sleep is very important.

Sun, Photons and Electrons

Sun, photons, electrons - What are they?

Sun rays reach the earth as an inexhaustible source of energy. The sources of power in mineral oil, coal, green plant-foods and fruits are based on the energy supplied by the sun's radiation. Light is the fastest traveler from star to star. There is nothing that travels faster than light. Light speeds along with time. Physicists emphasize that the photon, the quantum, the smallest component of the sun's rays is eternal. It is truly a life element. Life is impossible without the photon.

The photon is always in motion. Nothing can ever halt its motion. The photon is full of colors and can change its color, its frequency, when present in large numbers. The photon - acknowledged to be the purest form of energy, the purest wave, always in motion—can unite with a second photon, when it is in resonance with the other, to form a "short-lived particle." This particle, known as "O" particle, can break up into two photons again, without mass, as a pure wave in motion. This is the basis for the wonderful back and forth movement between light and matter. This photon can never be pinned down to one location. This is the foundation for the Theory of Relativity. The photon gave rise to Max Planck's and Einstein's formation of the quantum theory which is of such significance today.

Electrons

Electrons are a smallest particles of matter and are in continual movements. They vibrate continually on their own wavelength. They have their own frequency, like radio receivers which are set at a certain wavelength. The electron orbits in matter around a nucleus. The heavy matter in the nucleus (proton) is charged with positive electricity. In contrast to this, the electron carries a negative charge. The positively charged nucleus and the negatively charged electron attract each other by means of their electrical opposition. But the electron, always in motion, never approaches the nucleus close enough to be drawn out of its own orbit. It maintains a certain freedom of movement within its prescribed orbit.

The electron loves photons. It attracts photons by its magnetic field. When an electrical charge moves, it always produces a magnetic field. The moving photon also has a magnetic field. Both fields, the magnetic field of the electrons and the magnetic field of the photons attract each other when the wavelengths are in tune. The wave length of the photon—which the photon can change—must fit into the wavelength of the orbiting electron so that the orbit maintains a complete wavelength. This feature is extremely interesting in terms of its physical, biological and even philosophical consequences. Matter always has its own vibration, and so, of course, does the living body. The absorption of energy must correspond to one's own wavelength.

Sunbeams are very much in harmony with human. It is no coincidence that we love the sun. The quantum biologists say that the resonance in our body is so strongly tuned to the sun's energy that: There is nothing else on earth with a higher concentration of photons of the sun's energy than man. This concentration of the sun's energy with their highly suitable wavelengths is improved when we eat electron-rich food. The electrons attract the electromagnetic waves of sunbeams. Flax seed oil contain high amount of electrons which are on the wavelength of the sun's energy. Scientifically, these oils are even known as electron-rich essential highly unsaturated fats. *The famous Quantum Physicist Dessauer writes: If it were possible to increase' the concentration of solar electrons tenfold in this electron-rich unsaturated fats, then man would be able to live 10,000 years.*

The sun's energy and man as an antenna

Almost everyone knows what an antenna is. The marvelous science of Maxwell, the physicist, concerning electro-magnetic waves today are well-researched and of practical use. Famous examples are telegraphy, radio, television, microwave oven, cell phones and various applications of high-frequency technology in the manufacturing of electromagnets, the atom bomb and research into nuclear power as a source of energy. Maxwell was able to show that an electric current flowing in an electrically conductive matter produces a magnetic field. Also electrically conductive matter which is moved within a magnet's field, will produce a current. When an atomic particle, such as an electron, is accelerated by an electric field, this produces electric and magnetic fields, which travel at right angles to each other, produces electromagnetic wave. These fundamental, elementary laws can also be applied to biological processes.

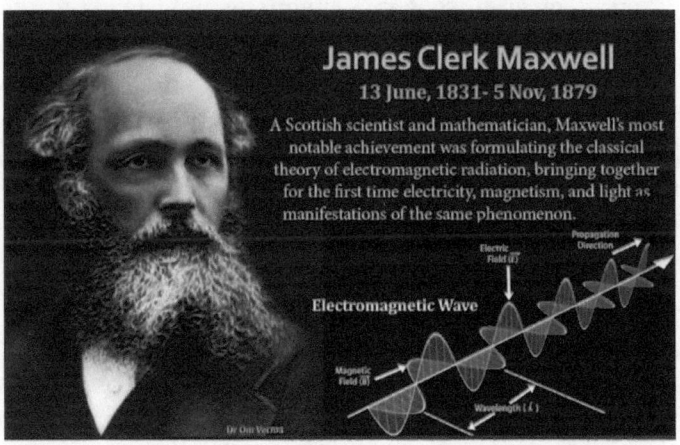

When the sun shines on the leafy canopy of a tree and is absorbed through photosynthesis, this causes movement in the electrical charge of the electrons. A magnetic field is also brought about when the water in trees rises. When we, with our wealth of electrons and conductive living substance, move through the electro-magnetic field of a forest, then a charging with solar electrons takes place in us. When our blood circulates, there is a movement of the electrical charge in the magnetic fields (for example, on the surface lipids of red blood corpuscles), which then causes much induction and re-induction of energy.

With each heartbeat, a dose of the body's own electron-rich, highly unsaturated fats from the lymph system, together with lymph fluid, goes into the blood vessels and thereby into the heart. This constantly stimulates and strengthens the electro-motoric functioning of the heart; Even the movement of the bloodstream is connected with radiation of electromagnetic waves-in accordance with the fundamental law of nature which governs electro-magnetic waves. This Transmitter within humans is always in action.

This Transmitter is also observed in neurons. The cylindrical structure of our nerves with the different layers and ganglions, with the difference in electrical potential between the neurons and dendrites, immediately supplies the picture of how strongly an electric current in a magnetic field leads to the emitting of electromagnetic waves. When I think a positive thought about another person, this involves the emitting of electromagnetic waves. The reception of thought also depends on the wavelength to which the receiver is tuned. There are amplifiers, as well as Transmitters that interfere. This encompasses a whole host of situations that are known under different names such as telepathy, hypnosis, mental telepathy, and many others.

Among Nordic peoples, it is known that the isolated native inhabitants use a tree to amplify thought Transmission, for example, to inform the husband who had gone to town, that he should bring back some salt. Bismark described how, during periods of trouble or pressure, he found relaxation by putting his arms around a tree and leaning his forehead against the trunk. In both cases, it involves electromagnetic waves that behave in accord with Maxwell's mathematical equations.

Fats Syndrome

The special relationship between photons, electrons and Essential Fats (EFAs) described by Dr. Budwig is due to the amazing molecular structures of LA (cis-linoleic acid) and ALA (cis-linolenic acid). The cis-configuration allows de-localized

180

electron clouds (pi-electrons) to collect in the bend produced on the chain. The resulting electrostatic force enables the EFAs to capture oxygen molecules and hold proteins within cell membranes. Like static electricity in a capacitor these charges can produce measurable bioelectric currents essential to nerve, muscle, heart and membrane functions. EFAs are extremely important to the body's overall energy exchange potential — the flow of life force.

Let us concentrate on the actual fats syndrome with its effects on the brain and nerve functions, the organs of the senses, the secretion of mucous, the functioning of the stomach and intestinal tract, liver, gall bladder and kidneys, the lymph and blood vessels, the skin, respiration, the immunity system, the fertilization processes and sexuality. All of these systems and processes of the human being are very much connected with electron-rich highly unsaturated fats, as receivers, amplifiers and Transmitters of electro-magnetic waves, and as supervisor of the vital functions. *The famous Quantum Physicist Dessauer writes: If it were possible to increase the concentration of solar electrons tenfold in this electron-rich unsaturated fat molecule, then man would be able to live 10,000 years.*

Anti-Mensch

Physicists interpret from mathematical formulae that man, with his wealth of electrons, is directed forward in time, which conceals within him the greatest potential to attract the sun's energy, and is directed against entropy. By means of these mathematical formulae, applied to Physics, and by reversing time, the mirror image of human beings is coined—the "Anti-Mensch", lacking electrons, lacks power and strength and directed into the past. It increases the occurrence of cancer. His thought processes, too—is paralyzed, because the element of life, the sun-attuned electrons, is missing.

The process by which x-rays, gamma rays, atom bombs or cobalt rays are set in motion is also equally directed toward the development of the "Anti-Mensch". The electronic structure of

181

the vital functions is destroyed by such rays. According to Feynman's "World Line Diagram" and modern theory of relativity, time and space have been given a relationship in a formula. The "Anti-Mensch" is directed into the past. Human's body tissues with its interplay between solar energy photons and large number of electrons, with its concentration of photons in life's activities and in the dynamics of the vital functions, are directed into the future.

But, when people began to hydrogenate the oils to increase their shelf-life; no-one thought about the consequences of this. In this process these vitally important electrons were destroyed. During hydrogenation, vegetable oils are reacted with hydrogen gas at high temperature. A nickel is used to speed up the reaction and unsaturated fats are hardened. This negative aspect concerning the development of the "Anti-Mensch" is in accordance with Feynman's "World Line Diagram". I emphasize that it means the fats and oils which have had their electron structure destroyed serve, within time and space, to promote the development of the "Anti-Mensch".

The electrons as resonance system

The electrons in our food serve as the resonance system for the sun's energy. Their electro-magnetic field attracts the photons in sunlight. The physicist cannot imagine life without these active and vital photons. These photons, which are in resonance with the electrons in seed oils, are focused on the same wavelength as the sun's energy, serve the life element. This interplay of solar energy photons and the electrons in seed oils governs all the vital functions. Fats are the dominant factor for all the vital functions, according to Ivar Bang.

The electrons of highly unsaturated fats from seed oils, which are on the same wavelength as sunlight, are capable of drawing solar energy and storing it, then, upon demand, of activating it as the purest energy in the form of the electrons clouds, and making it available for the vital functions. All the vital functions are closely connected with membrane function.

The exchange of electrons, the distribution of energy in the whole organism is dependent on these membrane functions — in the nerve pathways, the brain, in every organ, the liver, gall bladder and pancreas in the stomach's mucous membrane and in the kidneys and intestinal tract. The controlling functions of these membranes with their electro-motoric power, is felt everywhere. This is also true for the respiratory functions, and in oxygen absorption and utilization. It also applies to cell division — to all normal growth processes. It is true for the catabolism of substance in the elimination processes taking place by way of the kidneys, intestinal tract and also for the growth of hair and nails, as well as for the development of young life in the womb. Most significant point is that it is this electronic energy that heals cancer. This turning point in the field of proven successful cancer therapy is only one aspect of much bigger picture of the Quantum Biology. A lot of mysteries and miracles have yet to be discovered by doing research in Quantum Biology.

How can we once more reach the peak of human development?

Freeing you from the influences and effects of radiation and from environmental factors which promote development into the "Anti-Mensch", seem important. These goals, set by the individual who chooses, or by the state and food industries with their organization and planning, should be to see that the food we eat consists of electron-rich nutrition. An electron-rich food intake which supplies us with the resonance system for the sun's energy, must once more achieve priority. Such food, as the life element, promotes our sun-attuned energy. This in turn promotes our development, in space and time, into the future. The entire self can then grow and continue to develop further until, in accordance with the laws of nature which govern light and life, the highest level of our being is achieved. *(Excerpted from Dr Johanna Budwig's book "Flax Oil as a True Aid Against Arthritis, Heart Infarction, Cancer and Other Diseases.")*

Daylight

Dr Budwig focused upon the importance of daylight to our health. It is not enough to absorb electrons only through food, but it is important that we feed ourselves so that our cells are able to absorb and process the light coming from the sun. The more sickly someone is, the sooner he is "in the house", which can be a catastrophic mistake. Especially when people are already in a very late stage of the illness, they are often not able to eat enough and good advice is then very difficult. In such cases, Dr Budwig advises to concentrate on the following three points:

- ELDI oils as whole body rubbings and if possible as enemas
- Only freshly squeezed juices and distributed as food throughout the day if possible the breakfast muesli in different variants
- Stay outside as much as possible

You will experience me to explain what to do next. I have been able to see in my life how Dr Budwig's theoretical considerations work when put to practice, if indeed, if they are consistently carried out. If you could experience such a case yourself, and how quickly it can be better for a seriously ill person, you can see Dr Budwig's words in a very different light.

But other great researchers had also dealt with the subject of light long before Dr Budwig. For example, the anthroposophist Rudolf Steiner wrote, about 50 years earlier that there is a fundamental being of our material existence of the earth, of which all materiality has come only through condensation. Every matter on earth is condensed light! There is nothing in material existence, which is something else than condensed light in some form. Wherever you go and feel matter, you have condensed light everywhere. Compressed light. Matter is light by its very nature. In as much as a man is a material being, he is woven of light. Rudolf Steiner and Dr Budwig have pointed out in their writings over and over again the importance of light and that we humans are now heliotropes, which need light and use light. But I have nowhere else than with Dr Budwig so clearly and understandably read, WHY this is and above all, how the charging of the life battery works and / or what importance mainly the linolenic acid or electron clouds play. Because it is so important, I would like to repeat here again: The sicklier someone is, the more he should be in the open." (Oil-Protein Diet by Lothar Hirneise)

Visualization - Path to wellness

The visualization is perhaps the most important tool to tap into the power of your imagination to help heal cancer, manage problems or rather achieve anything in your life. Learning to direct and control images in your mind can help you to relax. This may help to

- Relieve stress
- Control some of the symptoms caused by your cancer or cancer treatments
- Boost your immune system to help your body fight off infections and promote healing

Past   Future

---→

Whatever you see around yourself is just a vision in the beginning, For example the cup of coffee you are holding in your hands or the house in which you live today did not exist in the past. Not very long ago there was a thought in your mind that you want to construct a dream house for living. Then you made construction designs and all sort of workup. Our whole life runs on the rails of time and never turns back. This is our time line.

First of all understand that everything around us is just a thought, energy or a wave. It is significant to understand this. Then only you will believe that energy can be converted in to a matter. Just imagine that a hypnotist puts a coin on your palm and makes you believe that it is hot. You feel burning in your palm. You may even have blisters on your palm. Here the temperature of coin just changed through only.

If you have believed that certain thought can change the condition of your body within seconds. Then why not a good thought can heal your tumor. In many studies Visualization trainer Carl Simomton has proved that cancer patients live twice if they follow visualization technique systematically.

Lothar Hirneise, the student of Dr. Johanna Budwig, respects Carl's research too much except a few points. Simomton teaches his cancer patients to visualize that their white cells are attacking cancer cells and killing them. Lothar is against this school of thought. Because in this situation patient focuses on his tumor. But Lothar says that main problem is something else, tumor problem is secondary. Secondly patient thinks of a war with a cancer cell, while Lothar believes that cancer patient needs balance and harmony rather than thinking of a war.

Lothar has interviewed hundreds of cancer survivors and came to the conclusion that cancer patient avoids direct confrontation with his tumor, but wants to remain busy in dealing with healthy and happy future. Though every patient has different approach, but end is same, creating a happy future. Lothar admits that visualization is the single most important therapy in his so much talked about 3E Program. After all if we will not create a healthy future for us then who else will do.

Please, review your time line again and compare it with thought-matter line. You will notice that both lines travel in the same direction and never turn back. You can never change the direction of any line. So start now and create your own happy future yourself.

Thought   Matter
———————————————————————————————————➤

Past   Future
———————————————————————————————————➤

I am going to discuss Lothar's technique in detail, which he learned from Europe's famous Visualization trainers Jack Black from Glasgow. Jack has taught his Mind Store System to 50,000 people in last few years. He is consultant of many celebrities and several companies. Lothar recommends that every cancer patient should attend seminars of Jack Black or Klaus Partl. Klaus Partl is right hand of Lothar Hirneise and teaches visualization at his 3E Center in Germany.

Initially Cancer patient thinks that the most important job is to destroy tumor. If he gets rid of tumor then he can plan to take some holistic treatments e.g. visualization. This is very bad decision. It is very important to follow visualization techniques as a part of your tumor destruction program.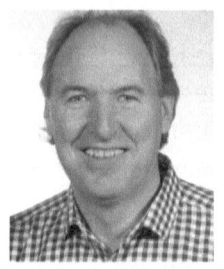

But How does it work? This word HOW is very important, because it usually prevents us to take right decisions. At this moment don't try to think how visualization shall work, how it is going to destroy your tumor. Time being I just say that try to trust us that it actually works.

In short I just say that you learn how to make your future healthy and cheerful, do not focus on present and past. Lothar says that if you know your past, it is easier to change your future. But your main focus should be to create happy future.

Your dream house where you heal your cancer

To give positive impact on your body and mind, it is very important that you become completely relaxed before you start thinking and visualizing. Relaxation or rather achieving alpha stage is the first step. Alpha means relaxed stage (7-14 hertz waves) of your mind. You can relate it with the alpha waves of an EEG tracing. Then there are beta, theta and delta waves. To reach this state there are many techniques or meditations. Some books and CDs are also available. Even listening classical music, meditation or mild yoga can relax you.

When you achieve deep relaxation, start thinking and visualizing. You start it by walking slowly along the right bank of a river. After a short distance you turn towards right. You see blue sky and green meadows. There are lot of trees and a very beautiful house with red terrace. (can imagine your dream house)

Now you enter this house. First room is a beautiful bathroom with a shower. You start taking shower. It washes out all your negativity, toxins and dis-eased cells. After taking shower you sit under the sun, the sunshine dries and fills you with energy within a couple of moments.

Now you go to screen room. On the blank wall of this room there are 3 big LCD monitors. You can relax on the comfortable sofa. You can control these screens with a remote control. On the side table of sofa there also lays a universal DVD recorder. Left screen shows your future, right one the past and the central screen shows your present.

Switch on the central screen, it shows your present sickness. Accept that many people suffered from this illness, you are not alone. Now switch on the right screen to see if you suffered from similar illness in the past. And if you suffered, then how did you treat it. Usually we don't find solution of current problems in the past. Now you minimize and freeze the past screen with remote control. Also, minimize and freeze the present screen.

Now relax and switch on future screen and try to find a solution to your problems. Now visualize a situation where you look perfectly healthy and your tumor has already dissolved. For example if you suffer from bone sarcoma in your thigh and can't even walk due to this illness; you may imagine that you are skiing in Switzerland. Feel the snow peaks, cold breezes, your friend's laughter, your own respiration sounds. Magnify these images, even increase brightness and contrast, and feel the reflection of these images on your body.

You may go to screen room daily, whenever you get time and see yourself skiing. Now you need not to view central and right screen any more. Directly start left screen, our next job is to record this skiing video on universal DVD recorder. The universal DVD recorder will relay this broadcast to the whole world. Your all nears and dears will know about your dream and start helping you to achieve this. To conclude the session, come out of the house and return to the river. Count up to seven and slowly open your eyes. Take a deep breath. This ends your visualization. Always keep in mind that the end should always be happy for everybody; nobody should be harmed any way.

Renovate your dream house if needed

You can construct some extra rooms in this house, if there is a need. For example you can make a small room for rest and relaxation. If you have some pain then you go to this room to relax for a while. You can also make a meeting room. You can invite here some important person to discuss your problem. For example you can call Dr. Johanna Budwig. You can sit with her, discuss and ask her opinion to solve your problem.

You can also invite your friends and close relatives to celebrate your successful skiing expedition. Imagine you are standing on the dice and narrating your experiences and everybody is clapping. The main essence of the story is that in the end people see you are healthy and cheerful. So that they also help you achieve your healthy and happy future. One question is very frequently asked is that how many times you should go to this house. Lothar says that there is no fixed rule but whenever you get time you should visit this house, may be twice a day. If the problem is serious then it is better you go there several times a day

Visualization wonderfully brings positive changes in your health. It costs nothing but works 100%. You can use this treatment to heal your cancer, make your life happy and cheerful or even to just become a millionaire (Hirneise, 530).

Unresolved trauma or shock

An important cause of cancer

Germany's famous Surgeon and Cancer Specialist Dr. Ryke Geerd Hamer was studying psychological aspects of cancer and treatment since ten years. He examined and tested over 40,000 cancer patients. He was amazed that why cancer of an organ does not spread to neighboring organ, e.g. he never saw cancer cervix and cancer uterus in a same patient. He also noted that each of his cancer patients suffered a psychological stress or shock during last 3 to 5 years prior to diagnosis and he was not able to come out of that trauma.

Each patient of Dr. Hamer also underwent CT scan of the head and in all cases he noticed some dark shadow or concentric circles somewhere in the brain. These dark circles would be in exactly the same place in the brain for the particular types of cancer. There was also a 100% correlation between the location of dark circles in the brain, the location of the cancer in the body and the specific type of unresolved conflict. It was very astonishing. Opponent radiologists said that the spots in the CT scans were machine errors (Artifacts). But Siemens Company which made the machine also admitted that these spots are not Artifacts (Hamer).

Thus Dr. Hamer concludes that when we are in a stressful conflict which is not resolved, the emotional reflex center in the brain which corresponds to the experienced emotion (e.g. anger, frustration, grief) will slowly break down. Each of these emotional centers are also connected to a specific organ. When a centre breaks down, it starts sending wrong signals to the organ it controls, resulting in the formation of deformed cells in the tissues, cancer cells. He also suggests that metastasis is not the SAME cancer spreading. It is the result of new conflicts that

191

might be brought upon by the very stress of cancer diagnosis or of invasive and painful therapies.

Dr. Hamer started to give psychotherapy to his patients along with the treatment. He felt that as soon as psychotherapy shows its effect, the patient is out of this shock (Psychosomatic), cancer cells stop multiplying and the dark circles of brain start to disappear instantly. X-rays of the brain now showed a healing edema around the damaged emotional centre as the brain tissue began to repair the affected point. There was once again normal communication between brain and body. A similar healing edema could also be seen around the now inactive cancer tissue. Eventually, the cancer would become encapsulated, discharged or dealt with by the natural action of the body. Diseased tissue would disappear and normal tissue would then again appear.

Breast Cancer always follows Psychological Trauma

The research from Dr. R.G. Hamer shows us that there are two kinds of breast cancer. We have breast gland cancer and we also have milk duct (intra-ductal) cancer. Each of these cancers has its origins in different areas of the brain and they each consist of different embryonic germ layers (histological formations).

Conflict Content

Breast gland cancer has its relay in the cerebellum and will form compact adenoid tumors that consist of the old mesodermal germ layer. Milk duct cancer has its relay in the cerebral cortex, (the sensory cortex to be more exact) will develop squamous epithelium carcinomas and is derived from the ectodermal germ layer.

These manifestations are in accordance with the rules of laterality. To be more precise, a right handed woman will respond with the left breast if she has a mother-child conflict or a daughter-mother conflict and will respond with the right breast if she has a partner conflict. Her partners include her life's partner as in husband, a friend, her brother, sister, her father, or even her business partner. The opposite breast will be affected in a left handed woman.

We do not develop either intra-ductal or breast gland cancer without reason. The specific nature or feeling behind the conflict will determine precisely what brain location will receive the impact of the conflict-shock (DHS) and whether it will be the duct or the gland affected.

Breast gland cancer has to do with the woman's nest in the sense that she has a "worry", "quarrel or argument" going on in her nest. The worry could be over a health concern of a loved one, or even being thrown out of the nest by her mother! The overall issue concerned however is really a separation from a loved one.

Milk duct cancer has quite specifically to do with the conflict of, "my child, mother, or partner has been torn from my breast!" Again it is a separation conflict and the rules of laterality also apply here.

Brain Location

As previously mentioned, each of these cancers have a different histological formation and have their relays in different brain locations.

Since breast gland cancer has its origin in the cerebellum, or old brain, the tissue starts to augment from the time of the onset of the actual conflict, and will stop growing as soon as the conflict has been resolved.

In contrast, intra-ductal cancer has its origin in the sensory cortex (cerebrum) or new brain and develops ulcers or cell degeneration in the squamous epithelial tissue of the milk duct during the conflict active phase. As soon as the conflict has been resolved, this tissue goes through the repair phase and begins to augment the squamous epithelial cells that will swell and eventually obstruct the milk duct and form a so called tumor. If the manifestation goes unnoticed, the so called tumor will either degrade or calcify and no longer be a concern.

In some cases the entire sensory cortex may be affected in the patient and she may display some very specific skin problems on the inside of her arm, hand, belly and inside leg, if there is a mother-child separation conflict. If she has a partner separation conflict, she could develop skin problems on the outside of her arm, or leg. The side of her body affected will depend on her laterality (left or right handedness).

The biological sense behind these manifestations has to do with where she may sit a child (on her lap), cradle the child (in her arms) according to her laterality, or where a partner is concerned, which side she may use to defend, slap, or push him or her away.

Metastasis

If a woman develops a self -devaluation conflict as a result of the original DHS that gave her the breast cancer, or as a result of perhaps a DHS she received with her diagnosis, her lymph glands will most probably also be affected.

The lymph glands originate yet again from another embryonic germ layer (new mesoderm) and therefore also have a completely different brain location for their relay. These tissues behave the same way as the tissue found in the milk ducts and will degenerate during the conflict activity and will regenerate or augment forming a tumor in the resolution phase of the self-devaluation conflict.

Naturally science has observed this and given it the label of "metastasis" for lack of explanation. However Dr. Hamer explains that if a different brain location and a different embryonic germ layer is responsible for the tumor, how can this possibly be observed as metastasis? He maintains that these primary germ layers cannot transform themselves into another germ layer once they are formed in the body.

So what causes metastasis? Dr. Hamer discovered that cancer is initiated by a DHS, (a conflict shock) therefore the progression of cancer or metastasis is dependent on further DHSs.

194

For example, the shock of having your breast amputated (a disfigurement conflict) can give you a skin cancer on the surgical scars, or a deep self-devaluation conflict (I am less than I was before) can cause bone cancer, the shock of the bone cancer diagnosis can give you a "death fright conflict" resulting in lung cancer because we believe that the cancer is spreading "like wildfire" throughout our body.

Metastasis in the conventional sense cannot exist in view of the discovery of the German New Medicine and the Five Biological Laws.

Testimonials of Budwig Protocol

Lucie Bois cured her Breast Cancer by Budwig

I shrunk a big tumor (8.5 cm) in my right breast using Essiac and Budwig protocol. Plus lots of fresh homemade veggies juices, organic products, coffee enemas and much more. You got to be committed to à very healthy lifestyle to heal safely.

The tumor has shrunk and could barely be detected on my last Doppler ultrasound test last September and my tumor markers went back into normal range. It took me 2 years and à half to be there. My only challenge now is cancer metastasized as Paget disease of the nipple. Long journey some would say. It would be too long to explain all the protocols I've used (and still using) just on a text. I could say that I used a quite big arsenal against cancer. Everything God has provided in His nature and non-toxic scientific methods. I never took chemotherapy, radiations or any surgery.

Prayer and my faith in à good God who wants the best for me. When you know that you are loved deeply by Creator of the universe who came on earth in the person of Jesus, it gives me assurance. I am also persuaded that God is very unpleased with the corruption in the actual medical system and is raising à squad of uncorrupt Ph.D. and survivors who will show à different way to heal while respecting the Law of Nature. Now I have a very good reason to heal. It is à mission. By Lucie Bois, Dec 15, 2016.

This testimonial is from my Face book group of 5000 members https://www.facebook.com/notes/budwig-protocol

Breast cancer healing reports involving Dr. Johanna Budwig's formula

Collected by Cliff Beckwith, a 15 year prostate cancer survivor "thanks to taking flaxseed oil and cottage cheese", and compiled and prefaced by Healing Cancer Naturally

196

Before starting to read the following healing testimonials, the reader's attention is drawn to these very important observations re breast and other cancer over-diagnosis and over-treatment as well as to the well-known power of the placebo effect as illustrated in these examples.

Breast Cancer Healing 1

Hello Mr. Beckwith:

I gave a copy of your testimony to a lady who had one breast removed and was given a grim diagnosis that the cancer had spread and that within a year she would likely be back to remove the other one. She had received all the chemo and radiation she could take.

The surgeon basically sent her home because there was nothing else they could do. She told me that she had no energy and that she had to give up all her activities. She believed that there was no hope and that it was just a matter of time.

She started the flax oil. For the first few days she felt more tired than ever. The fourth day she began to feel a surge of energy. She continued to feel stronger and stronger.

Within a couple of weeks she felt so good that she re-joined all the clubs and activities that she had to abandon before. She went on a trip to Eastern Canada that involved a lot of walking and said that she had no problems at all.

Two weeks ago she had an appointment with the surgeon and found that the other breast was fine and that she had no sign of problems. He told her to come back in a year for another check-up.

She phoned me yesterday to thank me again for the info that gave her life back. According to her, she was already taking vitamin supplements and good eating habits but it was the flax oil that made this miraculous difference. She said that she would continue to take the 5 tablespoons of flax oil in yogurt.

Andy

Breast cancer cure 2

A couple of years ago a friend of ours had a mammogram and it was suspicious. It was decided to do a biopsy in a couple of weeks and she immediately began using flaxseed oil and cottage cheese at the rate of three tablespoons of oil a day.

When the biopsy was done a malignancy was found. Other tests were done and a mastectomy was recommended. At this point she would have gone strictly with the flaxseed oil, but Tenncare would pay the $3000.00 for the tests only if she did what was recommended. The operation was set up but was postponed six weeks to try to get a surgeon to do reconstructive surgery at the same time.

It couldn't be worked out so finally, it was felt that she should have the procedure before any spread occurred. The operation was performed and the removed tissue sent to the lab for analysis.

There were no cancer cells detectable. She said the only good thing about it was that she had told the surgeon what she was doing and he suddenly got very interested because his wife had advanced breast cancer, had had a double mastectomy and was not doing well at all. He had had her flown to clinics wherever there seemed to be any hope and it hadn't helped.

The last I heard his wife is doing very well.

Breast cancer healing 3

A year ago last February through a real "coincidence" there were some tapes distributed at our prostate cancer support group meeting and one man was there who never came again.

That night he and his wife visited and she got flaxseed oil to get started.

She had had a mastectomy and there was a "bubble" that appeared. The doctor said it was a hematoma [blood trapped in tissues] and to pay no attention. The bubble was still there and larger a month later. She went to a different doctor and was waiting for his report.

Two nights later she called. He found it was a very rare, fast growing cancer. He gave her little time and no hope except possibly a stem cell transplant. She was in tears and angry that the original doctor had passed it off and wasted a month. She was now using the flaxseed oil and cottage cheese at six tablespoons a day.

When she had a checkup preparatory to the stem cell transplant the cancer had already disappeared. The doctor was mystified but told her he would guarantee it would return unless she did something else. He gave her something to boost her immune system and she became part of a study to test a new vaccine. They were aware that she was on the flaxseed oil. The last I knew sometime before Christmas 1999 she was doing fine and a friend and she were combining orders and staying on the flaxseed oil.

Breast Cancer Cure 4

In the summer of 1996 Debbie stopped to see us on her way home from her third chemo treatment for breast cancer. She had just gotten a tape and listened to it on her way to the doctor's. She wanted to try flaxseed oil and cottage cheese.

When she went for her fourth chemo treatment and the white count was done to see how low it was it was found that instead of going down the count had actually gone up. She took the next treatment, it had again gone up. She decided to discontinue the chemo and go with the flaxseed oil.

The doctor warned her against that course of action but she proceeded anyway.

The lump shrunk rapidly and she was excited. It did not disappear completely, but there has been no regrowth and she believes that what she can detect now is scar tissue. I have not heard from her for some time but I know she would call if there were any change. When I call her she answers the phone with "Praise The Lord".

Breast Cancer 5

In August of 1996 a lady who was a member of the church where one of my beekeeping friends attend had been found to have very advanced breast cancer that had metastasized to the bones. My friend gave her a tape and I called her one morning. She said she had been praying that she would be led as to the course of action to take.

The doctor wanted to give her chemo to shrink the cancer and then operate to prevent an eruption, but said it would not give her longer life or better quality of life. They did not give her but a few months in any event.

She refused the chemo and decided to go with flaxseed oil. The doctor was very upset and called her several times and urged her to follow his advice. The nurse told her she did not realize how ill she was. At this time she did not get out of the house on her own.

She started the oil and by late September was back in church playing the piano. I thought all was well and was excited for her. Then at Christmas time I heard she was in the hospital. We went to see her as soon as she got home and at that time she could only sit up in bed for a few minutes and was on hospice.

They had given her radiation to try to prevent pain in her spinal cord and it was not successful. They had not kept her warm enough and she got pneumonia. She told me she would never go back to the hospital again. She said they did something to her back that almost killed her.

Then I found out what had happened. She still used some oil after she felt better but stopped the protein. She hated cottage cheese. We got her started on Companion Nutrients.

The next I heard she had driven to the Easter Sunrise service and was driving to Knoxville. We stopped to see her a couple of times and she was mowing the lawn and caring for her garden. She said she still had problems but was improving.

Her daughter who was living with her told me that the hospice folks insisted on keeping her on a "pain patch" even though she didn't seem to have any pain by this time when it wasn't on for awhile. She said she didn't understand that.

Then she quit using the Companion Nutrients. She gradually went downhill and passed away.

At the funeral her daughter told me that the hospice nurse told her that when Emma Lee was sent home from the hospital that time the doctor told her [the nurse] that Emma Lee could not possibly last 30 days.

She lived over 22 months after that. One doctor told me that the material in the pain patch alone would damage her heart and liver if left on that period of time.

I wonder today if she had used the protein correctly with the flaxseed oil after she was back playing the piano in church if she would not still be with us. We can only go around once and we can't do it both ways.

Breast Cancer 6

Early last summer a teacher in a neighboring school district contacted us. A tape had been given to her husband.

This teacher had been fighting breast cancer with chemo and radiation for over seven years and was again in trouble. I do not know if a mastectomy had also been involved, but I don't think so.

They began using flaxseed oil with cottage cheese and she was doing very well the last I knew. Her husband used to come by for oil but they are now getting their own.

Breast Cancer ("her2/neu positive") Healing 7

Hi everybody,

I was diagnosed with a her2/neu positive breast lump, 7.5 cm, of which only a third could be removed, and not having all options available then, as I have now, started with chemo in January - what medical doctor, who we all turn to for help when ill, is going to advise you otherwise?

I had already had 3 treatments, lost all my body hair, got really ill and had my immune system affected adversely, when my dear sister in desperation started doing research on my behalf and came across the flaxseed oil/cottage cheese protocol and immediately started me on it.

At that time my cancer count was 78. When I had my next full blood count 3 weeks later before the next round of chemo, the count had come down to 43 !!!! I know it was the flaxoil/cottage cheese because before that, with just chemo, the count did not move at all. By the time I finished chemo, the count was on 23 and now, 2 months (stopped chemo) later is still coming down.

But now the very best news: a friend of mine developed breast cancer, had a mastectomy and had to undergo chemo as well. She was a bit hesitant to follow my advice and Not have chemo, so before she started chemo, I put her on flax oil/cottage cheese and my own supplementation programme and diet, which she followed religiously.

She started chemo -exactly the same as I had- adriamycin, traditional hair remover, included. She has now finished the treatment and to this day, HAS NOT LOST ONE SINGLE HAIR !!!! Also, was never nauseous, never had a mouth sore, never had a problem with low white blood count, and never got sick with so much as a cold right through our very cold winter this year. It was as if water was poured into her ! They cannot even measure her cancer -the count is so low!

202

Also, my Dad who also got lymph cancer this year -can you believe it, was also put on the flaxoil/cottage cheese diet and is now in remission! It's like a miracle. The huge lumps he had before are now just speckles on his scan and will soon disappear, I know.

All I can say is : IT WORKS !!! And I cannot thank my sister enough. My life is really back to normal because of her dedication and the flaxseed oil/cottage cheese she fed me! (am still taking it)

I eat it on fruit, jacket potatoes, in fruit shakes, as a dip with raw veggies, with organic honey on crackers. When you really feel you can't face it any more, just pinch your nose shut and swallow anyway!

Regards,

Lynette

The Budwig Diet quotes

"What she (Dr. Johanna Budwig) has demonstrated to my initial disbelief but lately, to my complete satisfaction in my practice is: CANCER IS EASILY CURABLE, the treatment is dietary/lifestyle, the response is immediate; the cancer cell is weak and vulnerable; the precise biochemical breakdown point was identified by her in 1951 and is specifically correctable, in vitro (test-tube) as well as in vivo (real)... "

Dr. Dan C. Roehm M.D. FACP (Oncologist and former cardiologist) in 1990

"Cancer patients suffer from a faulty metabolism caused by a malfunction in the lipid defense system. By repairing the lipid defense system the cancer cannot survive. Of course common chemo and radiation causes further harm to the lipid defense system -- the very system that protects you from cancer! The folks who will READILY ADMIT that they don't understand the cancer mechanism will tell you with their next breath that cancer can be killed with poisons. So can you. Would you trust your car to a so-called mechanic who didn't understand what makes a car work properly? If not, why would you let someone who doesn't understand cancer "fix" your body? The average cancer docs don't know - they admit it. That doesn't make them bad people; it just makes them unqualified to treat your condition if you have cancer. Don't let unqualified people poison you just because they don't know what else to do".

William Kelley Eidem, author "The Doctor Who Cures Cancer (Dr Revici)

"To sell chemotherapy as 'therapy' is most likely the biggest deceit in the history of medicine. Whoever masterminded this chemo-torture deserves a monument in the hell."

Dr. Ryke Geerd Hamer

"I have the answer to cancer, but American doctors won't listen. They come here and observe my methods and are impressed. Then they want to make a special deal so they can take it home and make a lot of money. I won't do it, so I'm blackballed in every country."

Dr Budwig

Dr Rudin believes the Omega 3 story parallels the story of Beriberi & Pellagra. It took them 200 years to accept pellagra was a nutrient deficiency.

"Nobody seemed to notice that a crime has been committed: It was the case of the missing nutrient. The nutrient was essential; it was a nutrient we human beings needed in order to stay healthy. It started to disappear from our diet about 75 years ago and now is almost gone. Only about 20% of the amount needed for human health and well-being remains. The nutrient is a fatty acid so important and so little understood that I call it "the nutritional missing link"….Food grade linseed oil & fish oil are the best sources of this special fat—Omega 3 essential fatty acid—which modern food destroys."

Donaldo Rudin, M.D. (The Omega 3 Phenomenon)

In a 1994 study of 121 women with breast cancer, those in more advanced stages whose breast cancer had spread to their lymph nodes showed the lowest levels of omega-3 fatty acids in the breast tissue. After 31 months, the 20 women who had developed metastases had significantly lower levels of these EFAs (Essential fatty acids) than those who didn't. Another study out of Boston University using the same type of tissue profiles that were used in the breast cancer study demonstrated that patients with coronary artery disease likewise had low levels of EFAs.

"The association between fats—meaning saturated, refined w6s (Omega 6), rancid fats, processed oils, and altered fats---and cancer, (but excluding w3s and fresh, natural, unrefined oils) has long been documented. (They) interfere with oxygen use in our

205

cells. Heat, hydrogenation, light, and oxygen produce chemically altered fat products that are toxic to our cells….These fats kill people. Healing fats in cancer include…… Omega 3s, enhance oxygen use in cells, decrease tumor formation, slow tumor growth, decrease tumor formation, decrease the spread of cancer cells (metastasis), and extend the patient's survival time. Unsaturated fatty acids in fresh, unheated oils are anti-mutagenic. Saturated fatty acids to not have this protective ability. Heating these oils above 150^0 C makes them lose their protective power, and they become mutation-causing. ALL mass market oils except virgin olive oil have undergone heating during deodorization…When we use virgin olive oil or other unrefined oils for sautéing; frying…we overheat them, destroying their protective, anti-mutagenic properties. ALL hydrogenated and partially hydrogenated products have also been overheated.."

Udo Erasmus (Fats That Heal, Fats That Kill)

"Our immune system, which is vital for destroying cancer cells, requires EFAs, vitamins C, B6, and A, and zinc to function, and requires an exceptionally rich nutrient supply of ALL essential nutrients for its high level of complex cellular activities. Deficiencies of EFAs and toxic, man-made synthetic drugs that interfere with essential fatty acid functions can create the conditions of fatty degeneration collectively known as cancer."

Udo Erasmus

"Compared to 100 years ago, Omega 3 is down 80%, B vitamins are estimated to be down to about 50% of the daily requirement. Vitamin B6 consumption may be low as it is removed in grain milling and not replaced. Vitamins B1, B2, B3 and E have also been lost in food processing. Minerals are depleted in a similar way. Fiber is down 75-80%. Ant nutrients have increased substantially---saturated fat, 100%; cholesterol, 50%; refined sugar nearly 1000%; salt up to 500%; and funny fat isomers nearly 1,000%."

Dr Rudin

Dr. Johanna Budwig is rightly known far beyond the borders of Germany. Her ingenious, simple, and effective oil-protein diet has found adherents throughout the world and it has helped many people to particularly better deal with their cancer illness.

I had the great good fortune of spending many days in discussion with her over a period of several years, of being able to study her extensive case histories, of giving joint presentations with her, and of thus gaining an understanding of nutrition for myself that extended far beyond that which I was previously able to find in the usual literature. But what was most convincing to me in my activity on the executive board of Menschen gegen Krebs in Germany was the oil-protein diet.

Hardly a day goes by when I do not talk with people on the phone that has changed their diet along the guidelines provided by Dr. Budwig. I am party first-hand to how successful this nutrition therapy is. I consciously use the term nutrition therapy and not cancer diet because I think it would be an injustice to Dr. Budwig to not to distinguish her scientifically grounded oil-protein therapy from all the diets that are offered around the world.

For me the oil-protein diet always serves as the basis of a cancer therapy and please understands that I am not just simply writing this, but that I have carefully chosen my words, as I have become familiar with more than 100 different alternative cancer therapies in recent years, and I have investigated many of them. When Dr. Johanna Budwig died the cancer scene lost one of the last great scientists of the last century, and it behooves each of us to carry her legacy to future generations, so that they as well can profit from the oil-protein diet.

Lothar Hirneise

I am referring to a super nutrient, which has been neglected for decades, it is neither taught properly in the schools, nor the doctors discuss about it openly, multinationals have removed this from our diet, but the hard truth is that it is essential for our body, it keeps us healthy and fit, protects us from many serious ailments, its presence is essential for cellular respiration, our cells suffocate in its absence, without this our life is impossible, name of this nutrient is alpha-linolenic acid, which is head of the omega-3 family and the richest food source is FLAX SEED OIL.

Dr. O.P. Verma, Flax Guru

They (American Cancer Society) lie like scoundrels.
M. Dean Burk PhD who worked for the National Cancer Institute for 34 years

There have been many cancer cures, and all have been ruthlessly and systematically suppressed with a Gestapo-like thoroughness by the cancer establishment.

Robert C. Atkins MD

Essiac Is A Cure For Cancer. I've seen it reverse and eliminate cancers at such a progressed state that nothing medical science currently has could have accomplished similar results. I wouldn't have believed it myself had I not seen it with my own eyes. I feel very strongly that Essiac is the single most beneficial treatment for cancer today.

C.A. Brusch, M.D., J.F.K's personal physician talking to radio talk show host and producer Elaine Alexander in a radio broadcast from Vancouver, British Columbia, in November 1984

The War Against Quackery is a carefully orchestrated, heavily endowed campaign sponsored by extremists holding positions of power in the orthodox hierarchy.....The multimillion-dollar campaign against quackery was never meant to root out incompetent doctors; it was, and is, designed specifically to destroy alternative medicine...The millions were raised and spent because orthodox medicine sees alternative, drugless medicine as a real threat to its economic power. And right they are...the majority of the drug houses will not survive.

208

Dr Atkins, M.D. (The Healing of Cancer by Barry Lynes)

And what do I actually do? I give cancer patients simple, natural foods. That is all. I take sick people out of the hospital, when it is said there that they do not have more than an hour or two left to live, that the scientifically attested diagnosis is at hand and that the patient is completely moribund. In most cases I can help even these patients quickly and conclusively.

Dr. Johanna Budwig, in "Flax Oil as a True Aid"

Cancer has only one prime cause. It is the replacement of normal oxygen respiration of the body's cells by an anaerobic (i.e., oxygen-deficient) cell respiration.

Dr. Otto Warburg, twice Nobel Laureate

...the cause of cancer is no longer a mystery; we know it occurs whenever any cell is denied 60% of its oxygen requirements.

Cancer, above all other diseases, has countless secondary causes. But, even for cancer, there is only one prime cause. Summarized in a few words, the prime cause of cancer is the replacement of the respiration of oxygen in normal body cells by a fermentation of sugar. All normal body cells meet their energy needs by respiration of oxygen, whereas cancer cells meet their energy needs in great part by fermentation. All normal body cells are thus obligate aerobes, whereas all cancer cells are partial anaerobes.

Dr. Otto Warburg Prime Cause and Prevention of Cancer

[C]hemotherapy is basically ineffective in the vast majority of cases in which it is given.

Ralph Moss, PhD, former Director of Information for Sloan Kettering Cancer Research Center

Three Australian oncologists - Associate Professor Graeme Morgan, Professor Robyn Ward and Dr. Michael Barton - undertook a meta-analysis aiming to determine the actual contribution of cytotoxic chemotherapy to survival in adult cancer patients. Their results, published in "Clinical Oncology" in 2004 under the title "The contribution of cytotoxic chemotherapy to 5-year survival in adult malignancies" (abstract available at www.ncbi.nlm.nih.gov/pubmed/15630849) found the overall contribution of these drugs to 5-year survival in adults to be an estimated 2.3% in Australia and 2.1% in the USA. See Table: Impact of cytotoxic chemotherapy on 5-year survival in American adults showing the percentage of 5-year survivors after chemotherapy for 22 types of cancer. The authors concluded that "it is clear that cytotoxic chemotherapy only makes a minor contribution to cancer survival".

A detailed review of this important paper is owed to Dr. Ralph Moss and can be read for instance at www.icnr.com/articles/ischemotherapyeffective.html under the title "How Effective Is Chemo Therapy?"

Healing Cancer Naturally

"Best book I've ever read on chemotherapy."

Ralph Moss' Questioning Chemotherapy is a book that every person faced with cancer must read before submitting to toxic chemicals which may very well destroy the body's immune system. Unlike many alternative health authors who base their conclusions on anecdotal evidence, Moss uses the medical establishment's own research to prove that in almost all instances chemotherapy is NOT a viable approach to improving cancer survival rates. Moss also makes the important point that current cancer research has never bothered to examine the mental anguish, physical suffering, and poor quality of life endured by almost everyone whose doctors talk or scare them into undergoing chemotherapy. Learning about the economics behind chemotherapy drives the final nail into the coffin of a "therapy" that educated people in the future will consider outrageous and reflective of the current dark ages of so-called modern medicine. This is a must read book for anyone who wants to know the truth behind chemotherapy or anyone whose doctor wants to inject toxic chemicals into their bloodstream.

Chet Day's review of "Questioning Chemotherapy: A Critique of the Use of Toxic Drugs in the Treatment of Cancer" by Ralph W. Moss

Except for two forms of cancer, chemotherapy does not cure. It tortures and may shorten life...

Dr. Candace Pert, Georgetown University

Chemo drugs are some of the most toxic substances ever designed to go into a human body, their effects are very serious, and are often the direct cause of death. Like the case of Jackie Onassis, who underwent chemo for one of the rare diseases in which it generally has some beneficial results: non-Hodgkin's lymphoma. She went into the hospital on Friday and was dead by Tuesday.

Dr. Tim O'Shea in TO THE CANCER PATIENT

Cancer researchers, medical journals, and the popular media all have contributed to a situation in which many people with common malignancies are being treated with drugs not known to be effective.

Dr. Martin Shapiro UCLA

~~**~~

Disclaimer

This book is not intended to replace the advice and/or care of a qualified health care professional. Please do not try to self diagnose or self treat any disease. Seek professional help and consult your physician before making any dietary changes.

This book is not intended to provide medical advice and is sold with the understanding that the publisher and the author have neither liability nor responsibility to any person or entity with respect to loss, damage or injury caused or alleged to be caused directly or indirectly by the information contained in this book or the use of any products mentioned. Readers should not use any of the product discussed in this book without the advice of a medical profession.

The Food and Drug Administration has not approved the use of any of the natural treatments discussed in this book. This book, and the information contained herein, has not been approved by the Food and the Drug Administration.

My Books

Cancer - Cause and Cure

Based on Quantum Physics developed by Dr. Johanna Budwig

http://www.amazon.com/Cancer-Quantum-Physics-developed-Johanna-ebook/dp/B00P3Y7BYG

Book Description

***** A must have book for every cancer patient *****

This book provides an introduction of Dr. Budwig's cancer research and treatment. Johanna

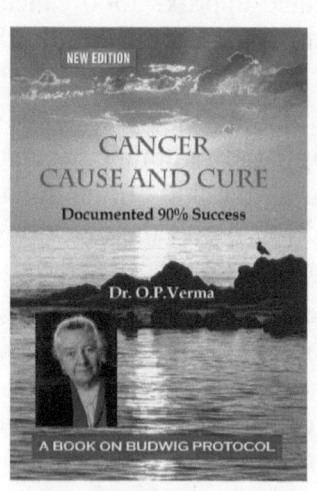

Budwig (1908-2003) was nominated for the Nobel Prize seven times. She was one of Germany's leading scientists of the 20th Century, a biochemist and cancer specialist with a special interest in essential fats.

Otto Warburg proved that prime cause of cancer oxygen-deficiency in the cells. In absence of oxygen cells ferment glucose to produce energy, lactic acid is formed as a byproduct of fermentation. He postulated that sulfur containing protein and some unknown fat is required to attract oxygen in the cell.

In 1951 Dr. Budwig developed Paper Chromatography to identify fats. With this technique she proved that electron rich highly unsaturated Linoleic and Linolenic fatty acids were the undiscovered mysterious decisive fats in respiratory enzyme function that Otto Warburg had been unable to find. She studied the electromagnetic function of pi-electrons of the linolenic acid

213

in the membranes of the microstructure of protoplasm, for all nerve function, secretions, mitosis, as well as cell break-down. This immediately caused lot of excitement in the scientific community. New doors could open in Cancer research. Hydrogenated fats, including all Trans fatty acids were proved as respiratory poisons.

Then Budwig decided to have human trials and gave flaxseed oil and quark to cancer patients. After three months, the patients began to improve in health and strength, the yellow green substance in their blood began to disappear, tumors gradually receded and at the same time the nutrients began to rise. This way Dr. Budwig had found a cure for cancer. It was a great victory and first milestone in the battle against cancer. Her treatment protocol is based on the consumption of flax seed oil with low fat cottage cheese, raw organic diet, mild exercise, and the healing powers of the sun. She treated approx. 2500 cancer patients during a 50 year period with this protocol till her death with over 90% documented success.

She was nominated 7 times for Nobel Prize but with a condition that she will use chemotherapy and radiotherapy with her protocol. They did not want to collapse the 200 billion dollar business over night. She always refused to support the damaging chemo and radio for the sake of humanity.

Lothar Hirneise is founder and President of People Against Cancer, Germany. He travels a lot in search of finding most successful alternative cancer therapies. He has been student of Dr. Johanna Budwig. He is a great researcher and writer on alternative healing. He is successfully treating thousands of cancer patients at his 3-E center in Germany. In the last few years he has interviewed several hundred final stage so-called survivors, meaning patients who were in the final stage of cancer and who are all healthy again today. Based on his findings he proposed a 3 E Program – The Mnemonic of Cancer Treatment.

1) Eat well
2) Eliminate

214

3) Energy

He noticed that 100% of all survivors, did the energy work. In approximately - say 80% of all patients, had changed their diet. And in at least 60% of all patients, took intensive detoxification rituals. This is the basis of his, so much talked about 3E Program for healing cancer.

Lothar Hirneise strongly supports holistic and spiritual approach and includes Visualization, Tumor Contract, Meditation, mild Yoga, Emotional Freedom Technique, Dr. Ryke Geerd Hammer's New German Medicine (Connection of unresolved stress and cancer), Detoxification techniques (Soda Bicarb bath, Epsom bath, Sauna, Colon Hydrotherapy, Coffee Enema etc.) in his 3 E Program.

The book also, describes about rare and miraculous herbs used in the treatment of Cancer like Turmeric, Black seed, Ginger, Mistle Toe, Aloe vera, Echinecea, Lobelia, Essiac Tea, Pau d'arco Tea, Dandelion, Milk Thistle.

~~**~~

Awesome Flax: A Book by Flax Guru

http://www.amazon.com/Awesome-Flax-Book-Guru-ebook/dp/B00PUUIR0K

Flax seed- Miraculous Anti-ageing Divine Food

What is Flax seed and how can it benefit me? I was faced with this question when I started hearing about Flax seed not long ago. It became a 'buzz word' in society and seems to be making great role in increased health for many. I wanted to join that wagon of wellness and so I researched until I felt satisfied that it could help me, too. Here are my findings.

Flax seeds are the hard, tiny seeds of Linum usitatissimum, the Flax plant, which has been widely used for thousands of years as a source of food and clothing. Flax seeds have become very popular recently, because they are a richest source of the Omega 3 essential fatty acid; also known as Alpha Linolenic Acid (ALA) and lignans. People in the new millennium may see Flax seed as an important new FOOD SUPER STAR. In fact, there's nobody who won't benefit by adding Flax seed to his or her diet. Even Gandhi wrote: "Wherever Flax seed becomes a regular food item among the people, there will be better health."

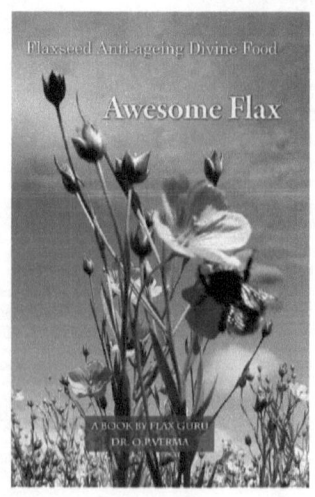

Flax seed contains 30-40% oil (including 36-50% alpha linolenic acid, 23-24% linoleic acid- Omega-6 fatty acids and oleic acids), mucilage (6%), protein (25%), Vitamin B group, lecithin, selenium, calcium, folate, magnesium, zinc, iron, carotene, sulfur, potassium, phosphorous, manganese, silicon, copper, nickel, molybdenum, chromium, and cobalt, vitamins A and E and all essential amino acids.

Other fatty acids, omega-6's, is abundant in vegetable oils such as corn, soybean, safflower, and sunflower oils as well as in the many processed foods made from these oils. Omega-6 fatty acids have stimulating, irritating and inflammatory effect while omega-3 fatty acids have calming and soothing effect on our body. Our bodies function best when our diets contain a well-balanced ratio of these fatty acids, meaning 1:1 to 4:1 of omega-6 and omega-3. But we typically eat 10 to 30 times more omega-6's than omega-3's, which is a prescription for trouble. This imbalance puts us at greater risk for a number of serious illnesses, including heart disease, cancer, stroke, and arthritis. As the most abundant plant source of omega-3 fatty acids, Flax seed helps restore balance and lets omega-3's do what they're best at: balancing the immune system, decreasing inflammation, and lowering some of the risk factors for heart disease.

One way that Omega 3 essential fatty acid known as Alpha Linolenic Acid ALA helps the heart is by decreasing the ability of platelets to clump together. Flax seed helps to lower high blood pressure, clears clogged coronaries, lowers high blood cholesterol, bad LDL cholesterol and triglyceride levels and raises good HDL cholesterol. It can relieve the symptoms of Diabetes Mellitus. It lowers blood sugar level. Flax seed help fight obesity. Adding Flax seed to foods creates a feeling of satiation. Furthermore, Flax seed stokes the metabolic processes in our cells. Much like a furnace, once stoked, the cells generate more heat and burn calories.

Flax seeds are the most abundant source of lignans. Lignans are plant-based compounds that can block estrogen activity in cells, reducing the risk of Breast, Uterus, Colon and Prostate cancers. According to the US Department of Agriculture, Flax seed contains 27 identifiable cancer preventative compounds. Lignans in Flax seeds are 200 to 800 times more than any other lignan source. Lignans are phytoestrogens, meaning that they are similar to but weaker than the estrogen that a woman's body produces naturally. Therefore, they may also help alleviate menopausal discomforts such as hot flashes and vaginal dryness. They are also antibacterial, antifungal, and antiviral.

Because they are high in dietary fiber, ground Flax seeds can help ease the passage of stools and thus relieve constipation, hemorrhoids and diverticular disease. Taken for inflammatory bowel disease, Flax seed can help to calm inflammation and repair any intestinal tract damage.

~~**~~

Secrets of Success: Smart way to success for every student

http://www.amazon.com/Secrets-Success-Smart-success-student-ebook/dp/B00Q3IIVAO/

Secrets of Success

Normally people think that memory, intelligence or learning ability is a God gift and it is not possible to further improve or increase the brain powers. We take it for granted that it will remain as it is gifted to us by God. But the truth is just opposite. Understand that as you go to gym for workout to develop your six pack abs, feed your body with muscle building food and get sharp sculpted body shape. Friends, believe me if muscle can be built and remodeled, then why not your brain's hardware and circuit boards. If you feed your brain with proper food it needs, follow simple instructions and take advantage of neurobics or mnemonics, you can immensely increase your brain's abilities.

We have tremendous powers locked inside our brains, but we are not using them to full extent. Dr. William James, considered the father of modern psychology, pointed out that "the average human being uses only 10 percent of his mental capacity." We still have to find out how much power or secrets are hidden in our brain.

Nowadays scientists have discovered mysterious techniques and nutrients to boost our brain powers. Today I shall raise curtains from all these secrets; I shall disclose all hidden tricks

218

and tips. Today you are going to learn how your CPU, the brain tightly packed in a bony cabinet, functions. I teach you how each component and microprocessors works and how the best insulation material can be prepared. I also disclose the right technique to sharpen your brain and to make you an intelligent and successful scholar.

Today you will learn how to crack every examination you face, solve every question, defeat every opponent and get highest possible marks. You are going to write new equation of education and success.

Friends new boundaries and horizon of success is ready to welcome you. Today we shall discuss in detail about some great nutrients and supplements to boost your memory, learning, imagination, creativity and concentration. If you follow our suggestions and apply simple tricks you achieve a successful personality. This short e-book is going to prove a turning point in your life. Wish you luck.

Cancer Cure Is Found: Letrile is the answer

https://www.amazon.com/Cancer-Cure-Found-Laetrile-answer/dp/1797710206/

CANCER CURE IS FOUND

During 1950, a biochemist Dr. Ernest T. Krebs Jr., isolated a new vitamin from bitter apricot kernel that he called 'B-17' or 'Laetrile'. He conducted further lab animal and culture experiments to conclude that laetrile would be effective in the treatment of cancer. He proposed that cancer was caused by a deficiency of Vitamin B 17 (Laetrile, Amygdaline). Laetrile is a concentrated and purified form of vitamin B17. After a lot of research, he had finally developed a specific protocol to treat cancer. Laetrile Therapy combines Laetrile with nutritional supplements and a healthy diet to create a potent treatment that fights cancer cells while helping to strengthen the body's immune system.

Vitamin B-17, which is present in several different foods, consists of a locked substance which comprises two units' glucose, one unit benzaldehyde and one unit cyanide. When B17 comes in contact with a cancer cell it is unlocked by a hormone found only in the cancer cell, and becomes a lethal chemical bomb which destroys the cancer cell. Healthy cells do not cause breakdown of B17. Cancer is unknown to people living in areas with food products rich in B-17, and the population lives to a remarkably high age. Apparently nature has provided us with an ingenious defense against cancer, and it is an ordinary nutrient in our food. These are, amongst others nuts, seeds, vegetables, and in particular apricot kernels.

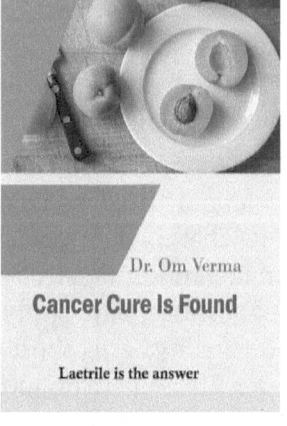

Dr. Om Verma

Cancer Cure Is Found

Laetrile is the answer

At present, patients listen or read a lot about Laetrile treatment, but usually they don't get precise and to the point information about what are the exact components of this protocol, where to get Laetrile injections and supplements, what to take, what not to take, what are the doses, how long to take the treatment, what diet they have to follow, etc. In this book, I have explained the protocol in detail proposed by Dr. Krebs. I have given every minute detail about Laetrile, other nutritional supplements and diet in this book. After reading this book patients can buy Laetrile injections, tablets and other nutritional supplements from the reliable sources (given in the book) and conduct the treatment under the supervision of their family doctor. Dr. Philip E. Binzel was personally trained by Dr. Ernest T. Kreb Jr. about everything of this treatment. Dr. Binzel had been using Laetrile therapy in the treatment of cancer patients since the mid 1970s. His record of success was astounding. Testimonies of his patients are also included in this book.